Acknowledgements

With thanks to all of my clients who shared their unique pressures, offered advice, played guinea pig and at times even proof-reading- you know who you are.

Thanks to my team for proof reading, fact checking and re-wording- without you I'm sure the facts in this book would be more invention than science.

Special thanks to my wife Christina, without her patience I would never have believed I could accumulate so many words in a row. Thank you for allowing me so many working holidays.

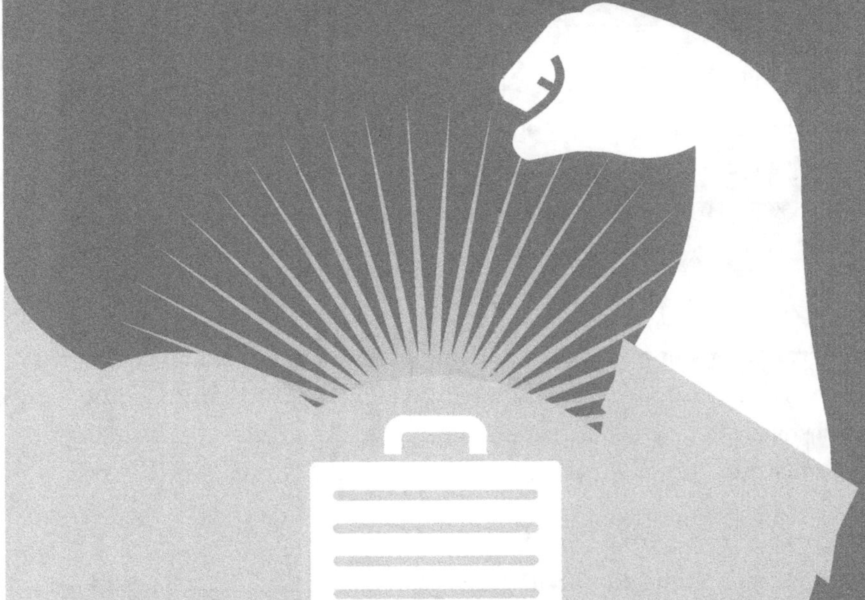

ED LEY

Contents

Chapter 5

Chapter 6

Disclaimer

Please note that the author of this instructional book is NOT RESPONSIBLE in any manner whatsoever for any injury that my result from practicing the techniques and/ or following the instructions given within. Resistance training can be dangerous if not practiced safely. If you're in doubt as to how to proceed or whether your practice is safe, consult with a trained personal trainer before beginning. Since the physical activities described herein may be too strenuous in nature for some readers, it is also essential that a physician be consulted prior to training.

For video demonstrations, coaching and accompanying pdfs and much more register for our exclusive members area over at

fitfor.biz

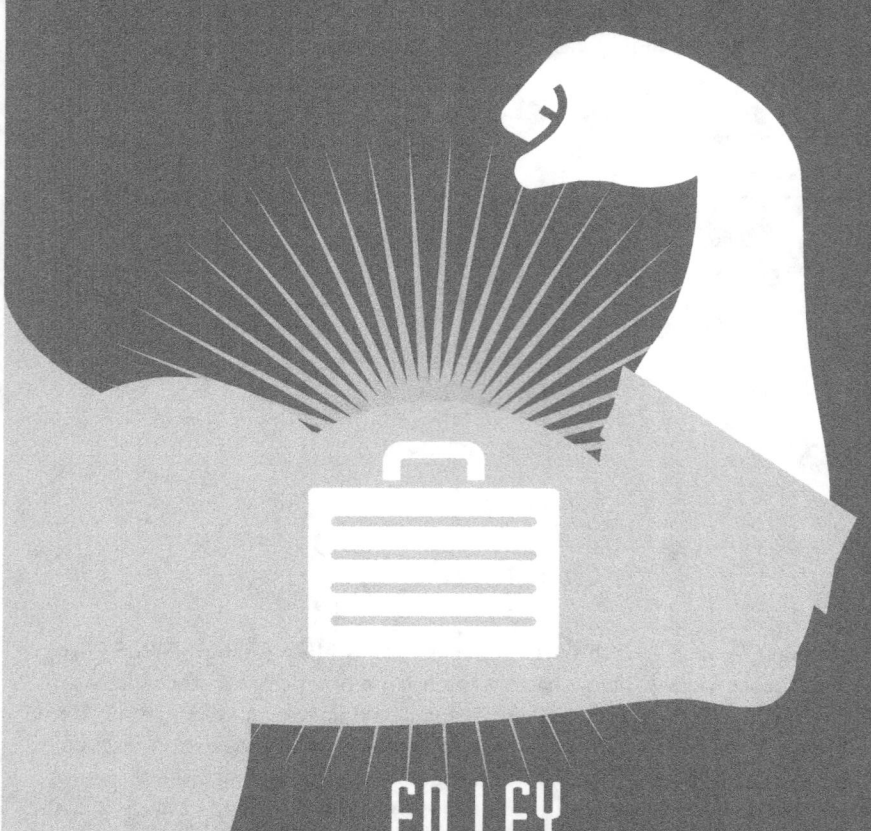

ED LEY

Introduction

'We don't see things as they are but as we are.'

Anaïs Nin

In my late teens and into my twenties it wasn't really clear to me in which direction my life was heading. I smoked, I drank more than a person should be able to without falling down a lot, and good nutrition could not have been further from my mind. I was not your model fitness professional.

Aside from the 20 hours of university lectures a week, my time was spent clubbing or in the comfortable environment of my local pub. I grew up in a small village just outside of Bristol, if you weren't in the pub, seeing your friends was pretty much impossible. Don't get me wrong, I was having the time of my life. If you had to pick someone out of the crowd who was there against their will, you wouldn't have chosen me!

When everyone around you is doing the same thing as you, your actions are very easy to justify and even to pass them off as the norm. 'I'm not as bad as some of them, at least I play football!'

It is said that we are the average of the five people we spend most of our time with. Health, wealth, intelligence, political opinion, relationships, motivation: everything! If you want to change something in your life dramatically, reviewing who you spend most of your time with is the quickest way to change. This sounds like quite a brutal process but it happens organically every day; meeting a new partner, changing your job, getting a promotion, joining a team or a gym, starting a new hobby, hiring a personal trainer, having a child. A number of events could completely change the direction of your life tomorrow.

While diet and exercise are tools that will facilitate a transformation in your physique and in your health, long term change requires more. Only when you are willing to look at your habits and their origin will you ever create lasting change. Changing my life required me to move away from my lifestyle. I'm still friends with those guys from the pub and you cannot blame other people for the course your life takes but, likewise, you cannot maintain a lifestyle of bad habits without negative health consequences.

The beginnings of performance engineering

My path into personal training, or performance coaching, couldn't be more textbook. Aside from all of my poor lifestyle decisions over the years, I'm basically a walking cliché! I loved sport at school and was pretty good at it (you seldom find someone good at something who hates it), so by extension I did GCSE PE which led to my studying Sports Science at college.

Following a year out spent working, drinking, not sleeping and trying everything the grown-ups told me to avoid, I decided to become a football coach. I found myself at university studying BSc Sports conditioning, coaching and rehabilitation. Quickly realising what a cold country I live in I knocked the idea of coaching on the head and turned my focus towards sports therapy, rehab and nutrition.

Throughout my time at university my best friend Tristan and I worked polishing Staples' shops' floors. We polished every store in the country. In order to do this, we would set off immediately after our last lecture sometimes driving as far as Sunderland.

The shops would close at 8pm and we would pour mild acid down on the floor and scrap up the previous eight layers of polish and then relay them throughout the night. After that we'd find a hotel, squeeze in a few hours' sleep and drive back in the morning.

With a day that consisted of an average 5 hours driving, 10 hours flooring, 5 hours lectures and 4 hours sleep my interest in performance engineering began.

My methods at this early stage were directed towards the necessary tasks. A very sensible place to start I'm sure you'll agree! First I looked at the 10 hour job; six four-litre tubs of acid, with 30% water added was cutting through eight layers of polish and creating one hell of a mess, yet only the top layer or two was covered in dirt. Two four-litre tubs with 60% water removed two layers; this made for much less of a clean-up job and only three layers of polish had to go back down. We were now in and out in four or five hours.

You're probably thinking; 'great, do half a job and you will probably be out in half the time!'

Well the end result was the same. The point of this story is that fairly often you can get 80%, if not 100%, of the results with significantly less effort, by simply reviewing your end goal. Our job was to make the store manager happy. A sparkling clean floor and five hours more in bed than he was expecting always did the trick.

From the relatively archaic beginnings of performance engineering with my advanced capabilities in cutting corners, my time is now spent helping people get the best performance out of themselves.

Through working with lawyers, accountants and IT entrepreneurs what I hear most often is more working hours equals more work done. When we look at this from an hour-to-hour angle, it's tough to argue. However, research suggests that performance drops significantly after just two nights of reduced sleep.

Reduced sleep is not the only thing that can cause a reduction in performance either: poor nutrition, lack of exercise, muscular pain and a number of other environmental factors all lead to a high percentage reduction in performance. From what I see, these factors are not the cautionary tale they are the norm. In business where your output is what separates you from the competition, you can gain the edge over everyone else without working more hours. You might even work less.

In a recent internal study at Deloitte in America, accountants working 16-hour days were forced to reduce their hour down to 12. Much to their surprise, productivity actually increased. The evidence of long hours affecting performance mounts up further still. A 1997 study into long working hours showed that even moderate levels of sleep deprivation resulted in effects similar, if not worse, than alcohol consumption.

Research shows the effect on performance of even a moderate level of fatigue is equivalent to or greater that what is considered acceptable for alcohol intoxication.

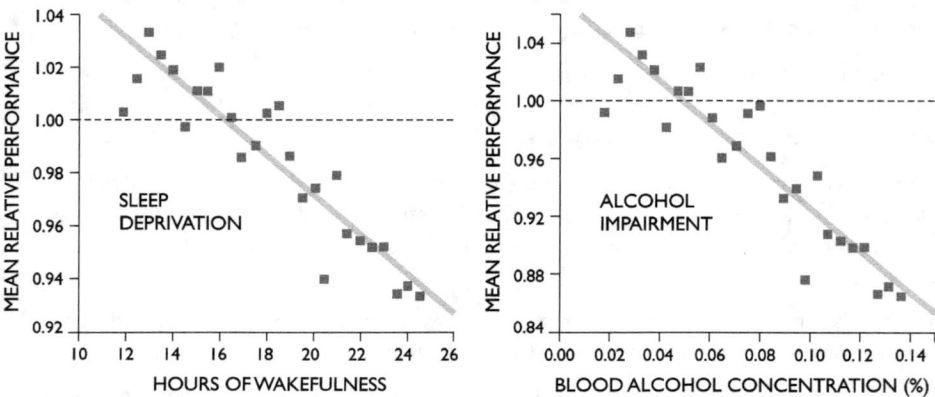

Source: Drew Dawson and Kathryn Reid's "Fatigue, Alchol and performance impairment," *Nature* Vol.388, July 1997

The impact of reduced sleep is easy to monitor but there are a number of controllable factors that can and do have a huge impact on your performance. Stress, back pain, weight gain, energy slumps, poor dietary choices, reduced sleep quality, loss of concentration, muscle loss, mood swings, anxiety, regular colds all affect performance and all have their base in stress, sleep, exercise and nutrition.

Given that the 'long hours industries' hold early and long retirements as a major goal, it pays to consider cancer, heart disease, diabetes, strokes and auto-immune disease in your approach to life. All of these diseases are 21st century issues that are largely caused by environmental factors.

In 'Science' in 2002, Willett noted that 70 to 90% of the risk for diabetes, heart disease, cancer, and autoimmunity is due to environmental factors. The genes do not drive most chronic diseases. It is the environment. It is time we stop blaming our genes and focus on the 70% under the individual's control. That is the real solution to the health care crisis.

Performance engineering is about helping busy people to mitigate the long-term and short-term negative effects of long working hours, while boosting day-to-day health, vitality and productivity. This book is about using systems in conjunction with a diet that supports optimum genetic expression and brief but high-intensity exercise. The most difficult part is building the habits to begin with. This book will help you to do this.

Performance engineering

My favourite film is Limitless, it stars Bradley Cooper who plays a down on his luck writer; he runs into an old friend who gives him an experimental drug called NZT500. This drug clears the mind and enables him to draw on all of his knowledge and the correct knowledge for any given situation. It also enables accelerated learning and expert execution in both physical and mental tasks.

The film follows the story of the main character but refers to others who have taken the drug and followed different paths to success, kind of like a 'choose your own adventure'. Of course, things don't work out for the best for everyone in the film (but things seldom do in films!). However, in life we all get to be the main character and choose our own adventure.

A first glance at the quest to become limitless had me searching for skills it would be cool to master, like playing the guitar, a martial art, gymnastics or chess, I realised that this was more of a quest to find a hobby or, at best, the art of mastering new skills quickly. Both great things but not what I was after. Who has the time for new hobbies or to master new skills? Someone limitless, that's who. Someone who doesn't get energy slumps, someone who's ripped who doesn't spend hours in the gym, someone really healthy, someone without bad habits, someone extremely productive. That person could choose their own adventure.

I needed to establish a model, something to measure against, something to define where I was and what needed to be done in order to progress. I dug out my university psychology papers and found Maslow's hierarchy of needs, designed by Abraham Maslow in 1943 as a map of human motivation.

The theory is represented as a pyramid with physiological such as breathing, sleep, sex, homeostasis, food and excretion at the bottom; if this were written again I'm sure we would find exercise in there too, as well as stress management and the absence of pain. My theory is that in order to move on to areas such as safety, love, esteem and self-actualisation (areas that encompass our reason for working, relationships and achievement and up to creativity and problem solving), we must first address our physiology.

Maslow's Hierarchy

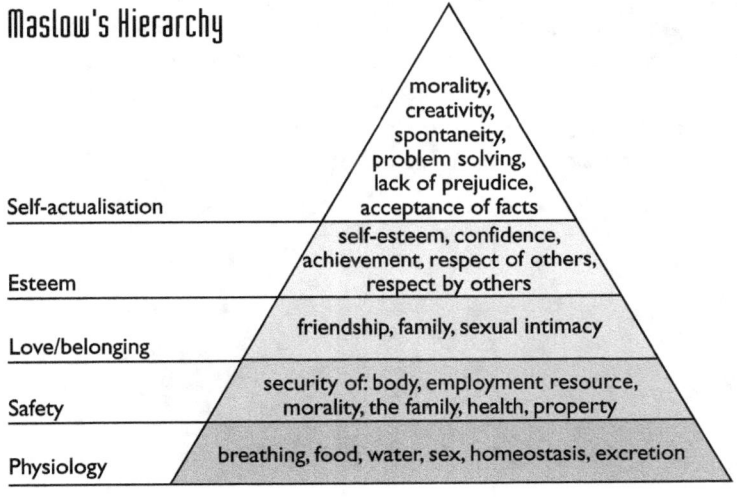

Self-actualisation	morality, creativity, spontaneity, problem solving, lack of prejudice, acceptance of facts
Esteem	self-esteem, confidence, achievement, respect of others, respect by others
Love/belonging	friendship, family, sexual intimacy
Safety	security of: body, employment resource, morality, the family, health, property
Physiology	breathing, food, water, sex, homeostasis, excretion

According to Maslow's hierarchy, physiological needs are the physical requirements for human survival and therefore the most powerful motivator. Without them, the body cannot function and will soon fail; we are genetically coded to seek these things above all else! I believe that the extent to which each physical requirement is fulfilled dramatically affects our potential in all other areas.

If we achieve only 50% of our physiological capacity, we only have access to 50% of the remainder of the pyramid; we will constantly be pulled back there each time one drops below 50%. Many of us spend too much time trying to move away from pain created by not fulfilling our physiological potential. Energy wasted on maintaining homeostasis takes away from our relationships, creativity and reasons for living as we define them. As humans, we spend our time focused directly on safety, love, esteem and self-actualisation and this is as it should be but, without first addressing our physiology, we will never reach our potential in these areas.

One thing in the world we cannot create more of is time and a huge amount of it is lost through illness, tiredness, physical pain, and lack of energy as well as the low state of performance that we all live through from day to day. This book is designed to help you create a habitual system that will enable you to focus on what is important to you for the rest of your life and achieve significantly greater levels of success because of it.

Ed's Heirarchy of Needs (2014)

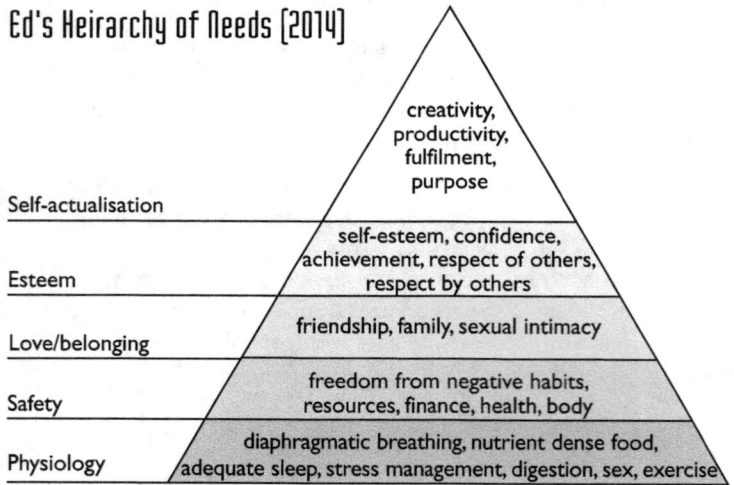

Follow the processes in this book and learn to master your physiology in order to leverage the best mental and physical performance available to you.

Chapter 1

You are the sum of your habits

We are the sum total of our habits. Habits are the things we do that require no thought process. Walking, writing, typing, brushing your teeth, making your breakfast, smoking - there was a time when you didn't or couldn't do any of these things. When you were learning to walk, it was your sole focus, you thought about almost nothing else. Eventually you mastered it and your brain made the skill of walking a habit. If you had to focus on the skill of walking every time you wanted to move, your mind would not be free to focus on other things, like the car driving towards you as you cross the road.

In short, habits are our brains making day-to-day activities almost involuntary. If you wanted to change the way you walked, you would have to focus on it every time you walked. This is true of any habit; changing a habit requires focus to remove in-built mechanisms and create new ones. We know that our brains are geared towards creating habits, so in time your new behaviour will become your new habit.

Success is one of the most frequently analysed behaviours in recent times. One often-touted attribute of the successful is their tenacity, not just because they keep going after many others have given up, but because they have a structure of daily rituals designed to bring results. Success is the result of repetition of behaviour.

We often believe that health and fitness are accessible only to the virtuous who are equipped with super-human willpower. However, health and fitness are best achieved with repetitive and habitual behaviour. By his own admission, Andre Agassi hated tennis with every fibre of his being but his pushy father forced him to hit 2,500 balls every day and he became one of the greatest tennis players in history. The point of this story is not that Agassi hated it, rather that, by the time he was 11, he knew of no other way to live.

If you weren't given healthy food and made to exercise frequently as a child, you are not going to find it as easy, but mastering the skill of health is accessible to anyone who can develop a repeatable process that is directed towards their goal.

Those who seem to have the answers now are often those who have the greatest number of good meals and bouts of exercise behind them. Their bodies and minds are simply repeating a learned behaviour. If this is all that separates the successful from the unsuccessful, then all that is required for permanent change is skill acquisition, simple repetition and an inspirational goal.

Habitual control

Our habits are a selection of actions that we thoughtlessly complete on a daily basis that make up the way we look in the mirror today. If every action we performed an on a daily basis required a conscious effort, we would never learn anything new and never be able to apply ourselves to any task. Every time we complete an action, a little less brain power is required to complete the task. Repeated frequently enough the action becomes automatic and we can focus on other things.

Forty percent of our daily activity is an automated response set in motion by waking up each morning. The key to lasting change is to discover what you are doing that you are barely aware of to sabotage your health.

The next step is removing that bad habit. By understanding how habits work, we can learn that most repeated behaviours are not addictions as much as they are the avoidance of disappointment. Once we experience a habit cue, our brain has a specific behavioural expectation. Habits or cravings are the result of our brains following an automated process designed to achieve a specific reward:

1. Cue

2. Routine

3. Reward

Once you understand this it becomes possible to change any habit.

When a habit is first created, a cue is set up to initiate the action. Brushing your teeth, for example; the cue here is getting out of bed, the routine is brushing and the reward is that minty fresh feeling when you're finished.

In *The Power of Habits* Charles Durigg explains that the minty fresh taste and the foam of toothpaste were added later and are not actually a requirement of toothpaste. These effects were however what caused teeth-brushing to become a worldwide overnight phenomenon.

The marketer may not have known it at the time but he had stumbled across the power of habits and was able to change the way the world worked as a result. His marketing message suggested that the white coating on our teeth first thing in the morning was disgusting and needed to be removed (cue). The only way to remove this coating was through brushing daily (routine). He then ensured that the toothpaste left us with a minty aftertaste (reward).

If we use this same system to look at sugar cravings, it is easy to see why so many people believe they are addicted.

Cue: It could be anything familiar and advertisers know this. That's why they always focus on making their advertising memorable. The cue is seeing the advertising or packaging of your favourite treat. Already a chain of emotions has been set into play that will result in you satisfying your craving.

Routine: Consuming the product or substitute product.

Reward: Sugar high.

Just like Pavlov's dog the cue is all that is required to prepare your brain for a sugar high and, when it doesn't arrive, you are left with feelings of disappointment.

When we are dieting we find it really hard work because we are constantly fighting this disappointment. The art of long-term success is in discovering a different routine that will produce the same result. This process does require focus and you will face disappointment until you find a replacement but, if you know your habit, you can change it. The important thing to know is that what you are craving is a chemical response within your brain. Any number of things could illicit the correct response you just need to find it. Fresh air, talking to a friend, eating some berries, 85% dark chocolate, exercise, music, reading: when you know your behaviours you can change them.

Use the chart below for a week to help isolate your bad habits and perhaps even isolate any feelings you are trying to move away from.

Discover your bad habits

What do you do? what do you eat or drink? how do you feel?	
24:00	
01:00	
02:00	
03:00	
04:00	
05:00	
06:00	
07:00	
08:00	
09:00	
10:00	
11:00	
12:00	
13:00	
14:00	
15:00	
16:00	
17:00	
18:00	
19:00	
20:00	
21:00	
22:00	
23:00	

Changing your habits

By now you have discovered your bad habits. The next step is to change them. Pick one and isolate your cue, routine and reward. And fill in the first part of the form. The aim now is to attempt a number of substitute routines until you are able to illicit the same reward feeling. This requires you to get creative. If we look at a 3pm cake as an example: it could be that you are experiencing a sugar low after lunch and changes in your diet will help with this, but the 3pm habit will still remain forever unless you change it.

It could be that not only are you experiencing a sugar low but also a mental low. Do you need to take a walk or a break from whatever you are working on? Are you looking to reward yourself for a hard day's work? You may need to eat something else. Everyone is different and experimentation and persistence will eventually yield results.

Use the chart below to practise substituting and to monitor how you feel until you get to the root of you habit:

1. Record your cue.

2. Record your substitute.

3. Record your reward (this won't change, if you get the substitute right).

4. Record how you feel one hour after you substitute.

5. Did it work?

Once you find a substitute any further attempts to change your lifestyle, weight or health will be far easier as they are less likely to be derailed by feelings of disappointment as a result of unsatisfied cravings.

Keep in mind that this process will not be an easy one. If your craving is strong and your substitute doesn't work then you will feel the disappointment. Not giving in to the disappointment will make you far more likely to be able to change your routine in the long-term.

Cue	Routine	Reward

Cue	Substitute routine	Reward	Feeling	Did it work?

Understanding ego depletion

Ego depletion is the force most often responsible for the beginning of the end of a new healthy regime. Understanding ego depletion is an important step in understanding why our willpower will fail to resist one day when that cue comes in.

Ego depletion is the tongue-in-cheek name given to the modern concept of willpower and all of the processes involved by Roy Baumeister and his colleagues in 1996. The name is a nod to Freud's theories of energy.

Freud's theory was that all mental processes survived on energy. It turns out that in the case of willpower he was at least, in part, correct.

Roy Baumeister and his colleagues designed a cruel study in order to ascertain whether willpower was depleted through its use. What better way to do this than with cookies and radishes, an experiment that plays right into the hands of a health book such as this one.

The experiment began by gathering 67 participants in a room filled with chocolate treats, cookies and with chocolate aromas. If you're thinking Willy Wonka you may well be going a bit far but, suffice to say, it was more than enough to get the 67 participants salivating!

And so the experiment began: a number of the participants were allowed to indulge, whilst others were left to satisfy their appetites with radishes. Progressing on to the second part of the trial, the participants were given an unsolvable puzzle designed to test their persistence.

The effects were clear; the radish eaters made fewer attempts at solving the puzzle and spent half the available time that both the cookie eaters and a later introduced control group persisted for.

Those who had to resist once no longer had the energy to apply to another difficult task.

This simple study highlighted a breakthrough in the world of psychology. Not only is willpower and self-control finite, it is also transportable across multiple tasks. The simple act of decision making depletes us of willpower.

What we learn from this is that our ability to resist temptation is most likely to strike at times of stress as we have less energy to resist. When a day's activities escalate beyond that of the norm we are more likely succumb to temptation. Although this could seem like something easily avoided, life will throw up different emotional, physical or mental challenges every day.

Any long-term lifestyle change is easier with an awareness of ego depletion and a commitment to habitual change.

Increase your willpower by forming habits

The brain takes up 25% of our caloric intake to function on a day-to-day basis. As food stores are depleted so too is our willpower. When willpower runs low our decision-making ability is hampered and we become more likely to act in a way that is not in line with our goals.

Even the most mundane of processes depletes willpower and this can have an impact on everything from marketing, to your staff, to how we treat people; and to health. Choosing what to wear in the morning, choosing your breakfast and choosing what work to focus on all have an impact on your willpower.

You may have tried sticking to something in the past and found that it was easier on days where most things were habitual. Holidays, weekends and any other interruption in the status quo increase the number of decisions we have to make on a daily basis and our willpower struggles to keep up.

On an average work day my routine starts as follows:

1. Get up.

2. Brush teeth.

3. Shower.

4. Eat breakfast.

5. Put on pre-laid-out clothes.

6. Cycle to work.

I have created a set of habits. I am an hour into my day and I have made no decisions. The more decisions you can remove from your day the more likely you are to be successful in achieving your goal. This works for anything, not just dieting but productivity in business and in relationships. The hardest decision we all make on a daily basis is the last one: getting off the sofa and in to bed.

Giving up smoking is not difficult because the chemicals are addictive (only for 24 hours), it is difficult because it is habitual. Change your habit and change your result. In order to make health and fitness habitual we need to create new habits, to remove old habits and - most importantly - remove decision-making from the process. This statement may seem tangential but, creating habits in every aspect of your life will make each part of your life more successful, and will make sticking to a lifestyle change more manageable.

Without creating habits for your whole life, your new health regime will only be the top of your list of priorities until something unexpected happens and your focus deviates. The more your new life can be integrated within your habits, the more likely you are to create lasting change.

The aim of this book is to help you to create a structured daily routine: the by-product of which will be reaching your health goals.

For video demonstrations, coaching and accompanying pdfs and much more register for our exclusive members area over at

fitfor.biz

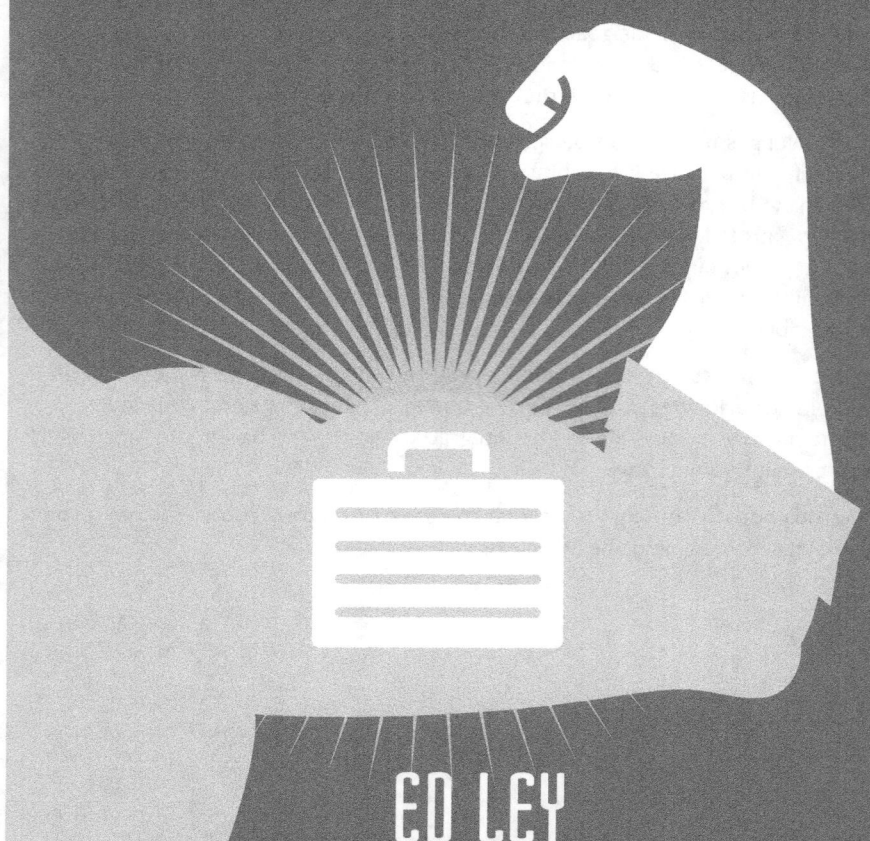

ED LEY

Chapter 2

Stress and the foundation for change

Every person is different: our genetics, life history and the way we interact with the world makes each of us unique. Constant external pressures from the working environment and from family life throw demands at our body that it is not designed to be able to manage. Each physical and mental demand placed on the body creates a flight or fight response. When we do not react accordingly chronic inflammation builds up, and this is the root of stress, muscular pain, poor health and chronic disease.

Stress - long thought of as a negative response - is the primitive process given to us to ensure survival, without which we would not be here today. In moments of stress, the body pumps hormones and neurochemicals into our bloodstream in order to activate physical and mental focus and memory.

This is most commonly known as the flight or fight response. Its purpose is to keep us alive and also to remember what caused the current situation in order to be more prepared in the future.

Unfortunately, our brains do not differentiate between good and bad stress: pressure to meet a deadline will elicit the same response as being promoted.

One major stress hormone dumped into our bloodstream during a flight or fight response is cortisol. During times of stress, cortisol takes over. It shuts down all non-essential systems and causes the body to produce glucose for energy. It will replenish energy stores and begin converting protein into glucose and store any unused fuel as fat around the belly. This cycle, when frequently repeated, is the cause of chronic stress and also the reason that doctors suggest that belly fat is one of the best measures of chronic disease risk.

Our bodies and brains are not the separate entities that they are believed to be. Stress and the memory of stress-provoking situations occur on a daily basis. A physical reaction is how our bodies are designed to deal with this stress. In order to maintain good health, we must give in to what we are evolutionarily designed to do, or suffer the consequences.

The human body and mind is designed to perform optimally when exposed to regular bouts of high intensity movement. Without it, problems we associate with stress and excess body fat can start to occur. Likewise, in order for the body to maintain good health and to function in an optimal way, its fuel must be clean and processable. A great deal of fuss is made about good nutrition and when we narrow down to specific foods it can become quite confusing.

The world provides clear evidence that, not only does dieting not work, but that no one diet suits everyone. Much like our bodies' flight or fight survival mechanism, our bodies have evolved to eat in a certain way and, when we try to change, our bodies and minds suffer.

The process of switching what you eat, however, is a far more complex process than the diet industry would have you believe. The way you were brought up to eat is habitual and difficult to change. A whole host of different hormonal responses have been set into place, often making our diet a product of trained behaviours.

There is also another evolutionary system in play. Our brains have no knowledge of today's abundance of food; our brains have only self-preservation in mind. Food cravings and our subsequent choices are a built-in response created by our brain's desire to survive and our habitual eating patterns.

In order to change the way you eat, you must first be aware of how you habitually eat and make steps to change that. Without changing your habits during times of stress, you will quickly revert back to your old ways.

The production of cortisol shuts down all unnecessary systems during times of stress, and making choices is one of those processes that is often shut down. Reverting back to your default habits is inevitable unless you break old ones and create new ones. If we are to live optimally, we must obey evolution and find ways to work with our bodies and not against them.

A diet or, better, 'healthy eating' cannot be a phase, it must be your norm. To change your weight, health, energy and stress, you must change the way you live forever. Maintaining a non-habit for the short term is achievable but maintaining a non-habit for the long term is impossible. Unless you commit to dietary and exercise change being a change for life, you are guaranteed to fail.

If you are anything like me, then you probably believe that you're different. Well, you're not. You cannot survive and thrive while also working in a high pressure job with long hours, alcohol, limited exercise and a poor diet.

Avoid creating a fetish

WeightWatchers, Slimming World and Rosemary Conley...these are seen as swear words within the health industry and that is not without reason; a focus simply on weighing less without a concern for health is a dangerous one. These programmes rely almost entirely on the system rather than the content.

These companies however are multimillion pound businesses; they must be doing something right. Perhaps we can take what is effective about these plans and apply a health and fitness focus to it. Many busy people turn to these programmes for help, they avoid focusing on exercise and they provide very simple guidelines.

All of the above have helped many people to achieve their weight loss goals yet they all advocate a very different approach to each other. They are all however the same in three areas:

1. They offer an easy-to-follow systematic approach.

2. They result in a caloric deficit.

3. They make no food off-limits.

Social media is great for shining a light on big problems without it always being obvious to those involved. I am a member of a number of groups on Facebook that discuss diet and exercise in great detail on a regular basis and a consensus is seldom reached.

I think that we often end up in a state of paralysis by analysis; over-thinking is perhaps the main reason that people fail or fail to get started in the first place. Successful businesses know this and they know that using a method that is 80% right, while following a structured plan and altering as you go is the best way to get the job done.

Starting any project with a detailed plan dramatically increases success rates in both the short-term and the long-term. In the short-term it helps you to override old habits and stay on track; in the long-term, it helps to create new habits. A diet, weight loss programme, health programme, toning programme; whatever you want to call it, needs to be viewed as a complete lifestyle change forever, not just until you get closer to the results you want.

Keeping one foot in your old life will make any change impossible, and may even be detrimental to your health. Fear of loss can often keep us attached to our current way of life but, without the willingness to let it go, long-term change is not possible. If you have intentions of leaving one foot in your current lifestyle, this plan isn't for you. Everything in moderation is a failed cliché, half following a plan just doesn't work. This isn't to suggest that you have to give up everything you love forever but, in order to change things for the long-term, you require a stream of early back-to-back successes.

Making no food off-limits is seen by the fitness industry as the greatest weakness of the big diet companies. A closer look, however, reveals that it is their greatest strength. Often seen as being a low barrier to entry, designed to keep its followers permanently in yo-yo, it is designed to avoid failure.

There are foods that you would do very well to cut out of your life altogether but, as soon as we are told to cut them out, we create a fetish. Don't think of a pink elephant.

Russell Brand demonstrated this concept perfectly in his latest stand-up:

'I think what I *meant* to say when during the MTV VMA Awards, I implied that the Jonas Brothers' chastity rings and virginity might in fact be a cynical marketing ploy, utilising the theories of Michel Foucault, who said that in Victorian society, the repression of sexuality was just another way of bringing sexuality to the forefront of our consciousnesses. It's a marketing technique. By saying that the Jonas brothers are virgins, you can't help but think about them having sex.'

By making food off-limits you guarantee eventual failure. By assigning consequences to foods that are not helpful to your weight-loss goals, these diets simply make avoiding the foods the wisest choice.

If you have 30 points worth of food available to you all day and a slice of bread takes up five you are likely to avoid it in favour of something worth fewer points so that you can eat more. This is a sound theory that works, as long as you follow the plan, and may even help to create long-term habits.

Whereas the plans will often work, some of them completely avoid health improvement making long-term weight-management impossible and our goal of improved performance just as impossible. And, equally as important, none of them empower you with education. They create dependence so that any change in circumstance will affect your progress and results.

The power of good stress

I had my father-in-law proof-read my first draft of this book and, as my target demographic, I had to listen when he posed the question: "What if you enjoy your job?" Had he been a little more patient, he would have made it to the nutrition section in which I discuss the "thrive or survive" concept of stress. Without giving too much away, most people find themselves in a survival mode trying to create change by adding additional stressors to their life. It seldom works. The body is focused on survival and when in survival mode, very little can change.

No doubt, you will have had a holiday in recent years where you were ill. You had worked hard for weeks, the deadline pressed right up to the last minute and you really deserved the break. Waking up with a brutal cold on the first day of your holiday was not part of your plan. Some people will report a similar phenomenon after a relaxing massage. The mechanism at work here is stress; sleeping shorter and keeping your brain alert for weeks or months on end has told your brain to be in survival mode. In survival mode, the brain releases cortisol, the stress hormone, which keeps us focused and vigilant to attack from wild beasts and the like. While vigilance is required, sickness is not helpful; the body shuts the immune system down.

When we go on holiday the immune system comes back online and - boom! - you get a cold. But it's not survival mode I want to discuss here, it's thrive mode where the magic happens. In thrive mode we have just enough stress to feed off it. There is one key requirement here: you need to love what you are doing. This requires purpose. If you don't love your job, or believe in what you are trying to build, no amount of health management will get you there.

All jobs have stressors and pressures that will, from time to time, leave us frustrated. The opportunity to vocalise these stressors is important - a spouse or a friend who you can talk to, or rather off-load onto, is reported to be of huge benefit. It is certainly my method of choice.

In an epidiomelogical study at the University of Pennsylvania that began in 1985, it was reported that those who believed that stress was a major factor in their health were right. The study involved 7,200 men and women. Those who believed that stress had been affecting their health "a lot or extremely" at baseline were more than twice as likely to die from coronary heart disease or suffer a non-fatal myocardial infarction. The study was adjusted to allow for lifestyle factors and the result was fascinating: 'whether you believe that stress affects your health or you believe it doesn't you're right.'

This doesn't necessarily mean that you can negate all of the negative effects of stress through belief but those people who believe stress is an important component in driving them forward are likely to enjoy the situation they find themselves in. A simple review of lifestyle factors is not an indicator of the impact that lifestyle will have on us.

Rather than pile up all of the stressors in your life and measure it on a stress scale, you simply need to answer this question: how much do you believe stress affects your health? If you answer a lot, you need to make a change in what you are doing or at least re-discover why you are doing it. In order to thrive, you must find meaning in what you are doing.

Awake Apnea

Breathing sits at the base of Maslow's Hierarchy as a fundamental motivator and it is obvious why - at a base level, if we don't breathe we die. You'd be forgiven for thinking that breathing was a given, if you're alive, you're breathing, but it turns out that the way we breathe can have a huge impact on our health. Email could be causing us bigger problems than wasting time.

Recently in the gym I was chatting with one of my trainers, who was sat reading on his iPad when suddenly he got the hiccups and, not for the first time, we half-jokingly called it awake apnea. The phenomenon intrigued me: why did he keep getting the hiccups?

Although there are a number of causes for hiccups, e.g. excess smoking, alcohol and a change in temperature, what was causing Ally, a non-smoking, infrequent alcohol drinker sat on the sofa reading, to hiccup so regularly while tweeting and reading?

A quick look on Wikipedia showed me that hiccups can in fact be brought on by stress. Much like smiling will quickly make us feel happier, shallow breathing puts our body into a flight or fight stress response. We are preparing ourselves to make a rapid response to potential danger.

The anticipation of email and social media and even just completing a thought while typing creates a shallow breathing effect that triggers a flight or fight response. As we learned earlier in this section, failing to respond to a flight or fight response with activity has its consequences.

Breathing is as habitual as it gets. Consequently, shallow and rapid breathers are almost always unaware of the condition. Shallow breathing is best indicated by an inflating of the chest rather than the stomach and often by breathing through the mouth.

You're no doubt wondering why it matters in what manner we get our air, whether it's in many breaths or few breaths, air is air, right? Well, apparently not. Dr David Anderson, specialist in salt, stress and breathing conducted a series of studies 40 years ago that are more relevant today than they have ever been.

Anderson discovered that, when combined with high salt intake, high stress causes high blood pressure in large mammals. He noted that this sensation was accompanied by inhibited or shallow breathing.

Hyperventilating or shallow breathing causes a drop in carbon dioxide (CO_2) below normal levels, lowering blood and oxygen supply to vital organs due to CO_2-induced vasoconstriction and suppressed Bohr Effect. Voluntary hyperventilation can cause tissue oxygen levels to drop to dangerously low levels leading to, for example, fainting due to brain hypoxia. This is the effect in the extreme but shallow breathing, breath-holding and hyperventilating triggers the sympathetic nervous system, in a 'fight or flight' response.

Wikipedia says: 'effects of this shallow breathing fight or flight reponse include anxiety disorders, asthma, hyperventilation, pneumonia, pulmonary edema, and shock. Anxiety, stress, and panic attacks'. The longer-term effects of this can be weight gain, obesity, heart disease and a whole host of other stress-related issues.

Linda Stone *Hi-Tech Industry Consultant; Former Executive at Apple Computer and Microsoft Corporation says:* 'The parasympathetic nervous system governs our sense of hunger and satiety, flow of saliva and digestive enzymes, the relaxation response, and many aspects of healthy organ function. Focusing on diaphragmatic breathing enables us to down regulate the sympathetic nervous system, which then causes the parasympathetic nervous system to become dominant.'

At birth we are diaphragmatic breathers but new habits are created in the face of external stimulus. It seems that this is a problem remedied simply by awareness of its happening. The next time you go to your email be aware of your breathing and you will quickly remedy what is possibly one of the greatest modern killers.

Diaphragmatic breathing:

1. Sit up straight (imagine a piece of string pulling you up from the top of your head), and relax your shoulders.

2. Place one hand flat on your stomach, below your belly button.

3. As you inhale, deeply, imagine you are breathing into the lower part of your stomach and force it to expand into your hand.

4. Ensure you breathe in through your nose and out through your mouth.

It can help and even be meditative to practise this for 15 minutes every day but at the very least be mindful of it whenever you are focused on tasks such as email, typing, talking on the phone or using social media.

For video demonstrations, coaching and accompanying pdfs and much more register for our exclusive members area over at

fitfor.biz

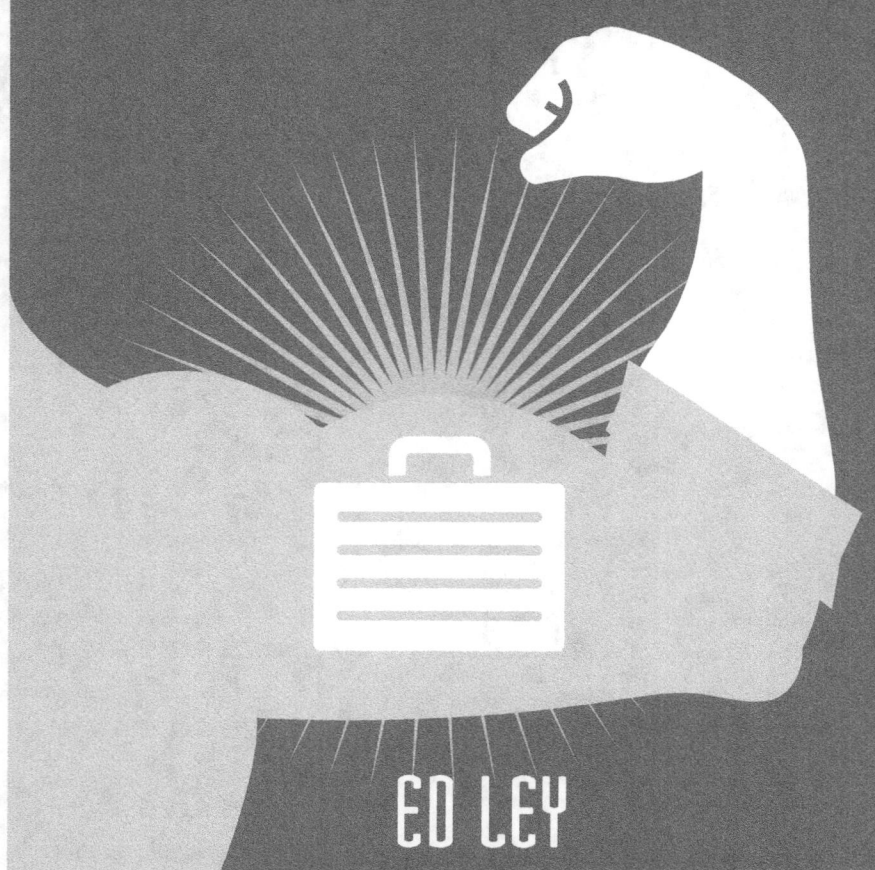

ED LEY

Chapter 3

The importance of sleep

I have read a lot of information on sleep. No doubt you have also read your fair share in the news. We all know that sleep is important. What I am trying to do with this book is to provide enough education so you feel like you have the facts and then provide some practical applications for improvement.

I work some fairly long hours myself; for me to get the recommended nine hours sleep per night, I would need to skip dinner and get straight into bed when I get home, fall asleep instantly and stay tucked up until morning. This is not always practical but hopefully there are some measures that you can take to improve just a little bit.

To highlight the importance of sleep, or perhaps provide you with some real world bench marks, I want to take you back a few thousand years. Like all mammals we are programmed. Our genes are built to support life in a world without electricity, houses, and modern convenience.

Our hormones and the way they operate our body's is a manifestation of two simple functions it is designed to perform:

1. Procreate.

2. Survive until we procreate.

Every response to stimulus be it exercise, sleep, or nutrition can be explained by this model.

We feel more alert during the summer because it's mating season. We feel wired, tired and like eating stodgy food in the winter because its hibernating season and we're still awake.

There are many other responses that should occur naturally; if they are not then something in your life is out of sync. A good place to start is libido. If sex drive has gone, then your very purpose for existing is compromised, which could be a good indicator that something needs to change. Men; you are meant to wake up erect. If women have no interest in sex then perhaps something isn't working as it should.

Testosterone is high both during and after a high intensity workout. Research has also shown that watching violent images or seeing a beautiful woman before resistance exercise increases testosterone and thus lifting capacity. Another study showed that if a woman sat on a man's knee when bench pressing Testosterone rose to 97%.

These studies support the idea that testosterone is evolutionarily designed to be produced to aid fighting off the competition during mating season. Likewise, the post cardiovascular exercise euphoria is similar to the feeling we experience after a roller coaster or a near death experience. Our brains have no idea that cardiovascular exercise is now a sport; it believes we are trying to outrun a lion and it's pretty pleased when we do. That feeling of elation is our body's method for encouraging us to do it again should the situation arise; which could explain why cardiovascular exercise is so addictive.

The book *Lights Out* by T.S Wiley and Bent Formby PH.D notes that as recently as 1910 the average adult was still getting 10 hours of sleep per night. In the 1990 we were down to 7 per night. The arrival of electric lighting and the subsequent reduction in sleep does seem to correlate nicely with the rise in obesity, type 2 diabetes, autoimmune disease, heart disease, cancer, and more.

I think the arrival of electric lighting would also correlate with an increase in manufacturing of processed food, longer working hours, and a reduction in manual labour. Sleep however clearly plays a huge part in the health equation. Of course that is all conjecture.

Fortunately, sleep is one of the most heavily researched areas in health. Of course it's not for sale so it perhaps doesn't get the media attention it should and pharmaceutical intervention has been shown to induce an unconscious state without the benefits of sleep attached.

Studies in sleep deprivation show an increase in inflammatory markers, brain shrinkage and an overall increase in mortality. All of which support the correlation with an increased risk of chronic disease that Wiley and Formby observed after 1910.

If we refer back to mammals' seasonal norms, our bodies are designed to be at a heightened state of awareness during the summer in order to procreate and fight off the competition. This continual state of stress can have a detrimental effect on the body which would ordinarily use the winters to wind down, store a bit of fat and recover. The arrival of electric lighting has put us into a perpetual state of summer or a perpetual state of stress. Our plan of attack could be to remove all electric lighting from our homes but this is a fairly radical step and one that you are unlikely to take.

Sleep, or lack of it, has a huge impact on every aspect of our lives. It is not just a measure of how tired we are but of how we respond to exercise, nutrition, fight disease, recover from illness, learn, retain information, look, feel and perform. I have battled with helping clients get more sleep for a number of years. Babies wake up in the night, deadlines demand longer working hours and quality time with our partners is missed. Pretty soon the only time you can get any time to relax is the time between 10 and midnight that we should be asleep.

Early to bed

The trouble with cautionary tales is that very few of us, myself included, are smart enough to learn from other peoples' mistakes. Very few of us think of ourselves as anything other than 21, and 21 year olds are immortal.

Chronic disease is for old people so at 21 we aren't really concerned with that, even doctors giving health advice can often be seen behind the surgery having a crafty cigarette; they're 21 too. Very few people do things to prevent something far off and intangible.

We are tricked into thinking that people change their bad habits because of the long term ramifications. We change because we are unhappy with something now, not something that might happen in 50 years time that happens to other people. This all makes sleep a tough sell, all of the cognitive studies into mental performance show that although mental performance does drop dramatically when just 1 hour of sleep is lost the body adapts very quickly. Mental performance doesn't improve but we feel fine. Unless we test ourselves regularly we are completely unaware that our performance has declined and thus we are unlikely to do anything about it.

Given that our objective is to boost performance, it is important that we remove this drop in it. Also given that almost everyone in the western world is sleep deprived, teenagers aside, getting the extra hour will put you ahead of the game.

In a 2008 study at Stanford university, elite swimmers were tested for speed and reaction time over a two week period. After the two week period the swimmers were asked to increase their sleep up to 10 hours:

After obtaining extra sleep, athletes swam a 15-meter sprint 0.51 seconds faster, reacted 0.15 seconds quicker off the blocks, improved turn time by 0.10 seconds and increased kick strokes by 5.0 kicks.

Mood and daytime sleepiness were also measured and showed a dramatic improvement with reports of much greater **energy levels**. Mathematically speaking, these increases in **athletic performance** are huge, and suggest that maintaining a good amount of sleep might be more beneficial to work performance than working longer hours in a sub-optimal state.

Research in 2011 discovered that the brain's empathetic sensitivity for evaluating human emotions declines when we do not get enough sleep and is in fact boosted when we nap in the middle of the day. Although I'm sure you might find napping difficult, if your job involves a large amount of human interaction and requires empathy then it will not only help to sleep more but to try and schedule your human interaction for earlier in the day.

Other studies show large boost in memory and creative problem solving when we are able to get sufficient sleep. Sleep deprivation is not as simple as just operating whilst tired, sleep loss results in a dramatic but personally undetectable drop in performance. Sufficient sleep is quite clearly one of the best ways of gaining an edge in business.

In case you were thinking about getting a weekend booster, a recent study involving Korean students found that getting more sleep at the weekend did very little to improve performance. Trying to catch up on sleep is like trying to catch a moving car on foot.

Studies show that the best quality sleep comes in the hours before 12, the earlier you can get to bed the better. Hopefully some of the tips in the following section will help you achieve the 7-9 hour target more regularly.

Circadian rhythm

Our circadian rhythm is the oscillation of physiological occurrences over a 24-hour period. All living organisms have a circadian rhythm. A recent Harvard study showed that healthy humans have a full cycle every 24 hours (approx).

If our circadian rhythm begins and ends with our falling asleep then the rhythm is the predetermined time at which physiological events happen, although as humans we tend to let free will act upon this a little more than we should.

Physiological events spread over 24 hours will look a bit like the diagram from Wikipedia opposite but are slightly different from person to person:

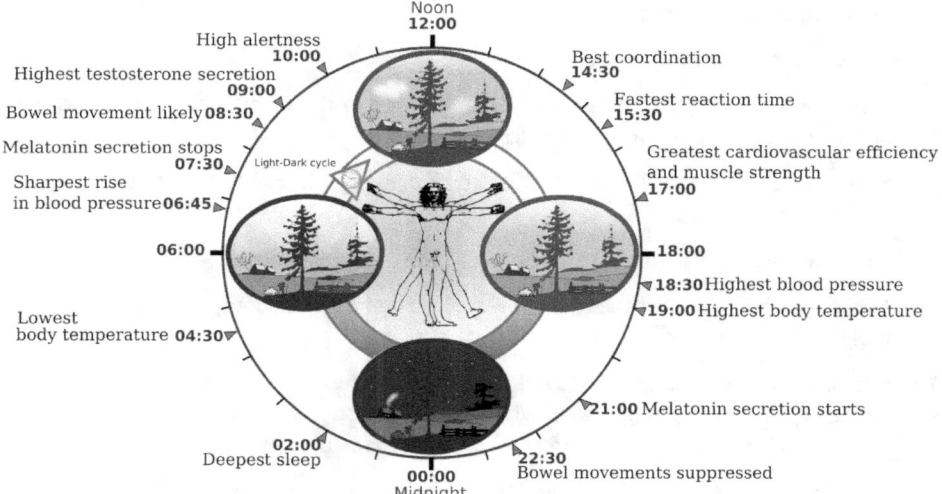

Noon
12:00

High alertness
10:00

Best coordination
14:30

Highest testosterone secretion
09:00

Fastest reaction time
15:30

Bowel movement likely 08:30

Melatonin secretion stops
07:30

Light-Dark cycle

Greatest cardiovascular efficiency
and muscle strength
17:00

Sharpest rise
in blood pressure 06:45

06:00

18:00

18:30 Highest blood pressure

19:00 Highest body temperature

Lowest
body temperature 04:30

21:00 Melatonin secretion starts

02:00
Deepest sleep

22:30
Bowel movements suppressed

00:00
Midnight

© The work was done with Inkscape by Yassine Mrabet. Informations were provided from "The Body Clock Guide to Better Health" by Michael Smolensky and Lynne Lamberg; Henry Holt and Company, Publishers (2000). Landscape was sampled from Open Clip Art Library (Ryan, Public domain). Vitruvian Man and the clock were sampled from Image: P human body.svg (GNU licence) and Image: Nuvola apps clock.png, respectively.

Discovering your circadian rhythm and living in sync with it could be a big step towards boosting performance. Discovering your circadian rhythm can be done using a blood test to measure melatonin levels. Melatonin being the hormone that helps us to sleep and continues to be secreted during the night, its production should stop to allow us to wake up in the morning. By discovering an individual's circadian rhythm doctors have been able to isolate the best times to perform surgery for optimum recovery.

By having an understanding of our circadian rhythm we are able to boast performance by improving our sleep quality, utilising optimum performance times and get back into cycle quickly. I have said already that catching up with sleep is akin to trying to catch a moving car on foot; trying to catch up sleep by pulling your bed time earlier than your circadian rhythm dictates can disrupt the whole cycle. It seems though that napping during the day has no impact of circadian rhythm. With that in mind it could pay to try and nap in the day rather than extend your sleep hours if you find yourself behind.

I have already mentioned that light has an impact on our sleep and this is true both for keeping us awake before bed and for messing up our circadian rhythm. Light and dark are what define our circadian rhythm; we are not awake as long in the winter as we are in the summer, or rather, we shouldn't be. When the sun goes down melatonin production is at its highest and sends us off to sleep. When the sun comes up production goes down and we get a cortisol boost to wake up us up.

Electric lighting in the evening and, worse still, in the middle of the night disrupts this process. Light exposure and turning on lights in the middle of the night signals to your body that it is morning. Melatonin production then slows, disrupting recovery from the days stressors and sleep quality.

Living as close as you can to the cycles of light and dark would deliver a huge boost to your health. The first step here is shutting out light.

1. Dark curtains or shutters.

2. Switch off all electrical appliances.

3. Don't switch on lights in the night (having to pee in the night is not a sign of aging but perhaps too much to drink before bed).

4. Switch off the TV and dim the lighting an hour before bed. Any efforts to darken surroundings will help.

5. Use low level lighting during the evening such as floor lamps.

6. Avoid looking into bright screens for during the last hour before sleep ie phone, tablet, computer or celevision.

You can also note consistency in bowel movement. If they are inconsistent then something is potentially going wrong with your digestion, this should be brought into line with the adjustment of circadian rhythm or perhaps dietary intervention.

Try and aim for the same bed time and wake time every day; if you miss it then try and nap rather than extend your next sleep cycle. If your circadian rhythm and sleep cycle is a complete mess then forced tiredness seems to be the best method for recovering it.

On night one of your sleep fixing cycle you should aim to say up until 2am and wake up at your normal wake up time. Then take your sleep I hour earlier each night until you feel a proper sleep cycle has been restored.

Creating a ritual

If you are fortunate enough to have a relatively consistent evening /bed time pattern it can help to create an evening ritual. Just like the structure of the morning when we brush our teeth, shower, have breakfast, get dressed etc the last hour or two before bed can often follow a habitual pattern.

The evening ritual, unlike the morning, has two things that may throw us off course: ego depletion and a reduced sense of urgency. A later bedtime has a seemingly less harsh punishment than being late for work. Although, it could, arguably, have a much greater impact on work performance. Still I think we are safe from our employers dictating our bed time for the time being.

The reduction in urgency and often the introduction of the television means that although we have an evening ritual the time it ends often depends on when our favourite programme finishes.

Ask yourself what needs to happen in order for you to get a good night's sleep?

We already know we need to create darkness and we need to swap overhead lighting for low level lighting. The next step is to create an environment in which you physically and mental relax while letting your brain and body know it is time to start preparing for sleep.

For me mental relaxation means turning off email while also keeping a pad to hand in case I need to write something down to remember for the morning. It means preparing what I am going to wear to work or need to take to work the next day. Whatever being ready for tomorrow means to you make sure you get it done before your evening ritual beings. It could even mean washing up/loading dishwasher. Try not to start your next day fixing what should have been done yesterday. Here is a loose guide for a bed time ritual but you can create your own:

1.   9:15pm turn off TV if its on and read book.

2.   10.30pm in bed.

3.   10:15pm brush teeth.

4.   10.00pm A cup of camomile (very relaxing).

5.   9:30pm Magnesium Citrate (helps your muscle relax).

*a great way to avoid getting sucked into the next tv programme is to record everything you want to watch and watch it another night, it also helps with avoiding the adverts.

For video demonstrations, coaching and
accompanying pdfs and much more
register for our exclusive members area over at

fitfor.biz

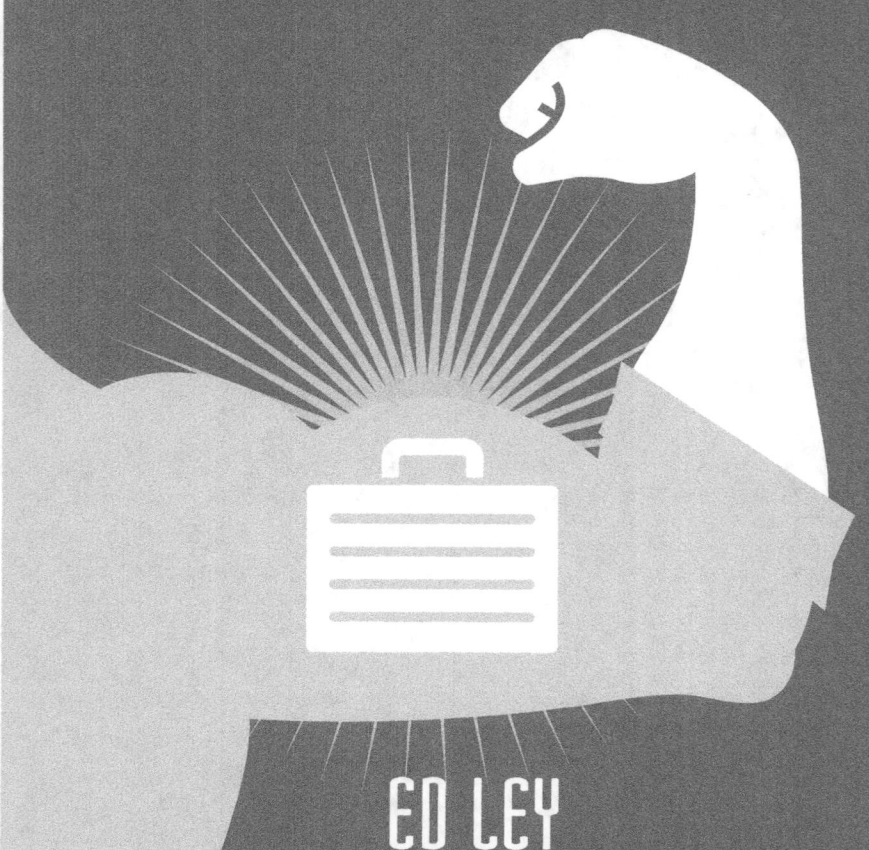

ED LEY

Chapter 4

An uncomplicated guide to nutrition

Survive or Thrive

Picture for a minute your stress levels as a bucket. Perhaps one like this…

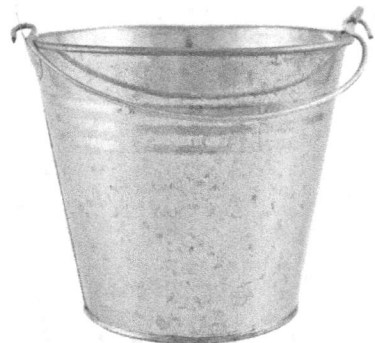

As I mentioned earlier, we require a degree of stress in order to drive us to succeed. Consider your bucket one-third full. No doubt you will have heard of or used the term yourself 'thrive under pressure'. As I demonstrated earlier it is important that we have this mind-set in order to thrive.

Too much stress, however, can push us into survival mode and it is often this that pushes us to change. Many people are driven to exercise and diet by not being happy with their current situation. For example, let's say you are overweight and keen to regain control of your body and your mind. A desire to change is triggered by a degree of discontent with your current state.

There are a number of lifestyle factors that will have brought you to this current state. So, back to the bucket analogy. It begins hopefully around 1/3 full and, in this state, you are in thrive mode. But to reach your current state there is likely more than this going on.

Financial pressures, home pressures, work pressures, reduced sleep, physiological issues, poor diet, lack of exercise, physical pain and a desire to please those around you all equate to an increase in stress levels. All of these contribute to your current emotional state and your bucket can become full very quickly. When your bucket is full your body is in a state of hyper-alertness. It is in full survival mode, your immune system is in shut-down and you are ready to defend yourself 24/7.

An attempt to change your diet and exercise at this time must be done very carefully if you are to avoid falling deeper into survival mode. Reducing your calorie intake now will tell your body that there is not enough food available. This means it is in your body's best interest to remain small and fat. It doesn't care how much muscle you have but it wants to hold onto body fat in order to survive the potentially leaner times ahead. Your body's primary goal is to survive in order to continue its genetic line. It reacts by reducing its energy requirements and holding onto body fat and burning muscle helps it to do this.

If you throw intense cardiovascular exercise into the mix and your body starts to believe you are being chased, it thinks you are literally running for your life. The feel good factor that accompanies your efforts is not a happy coincidence. It is your body incentivising you to repeat this behaviour the next time you are chased in a bid to live to survive and procreate. In this state you are destined only for disappointment. You are not dropping fat you are dropping muscle. Your brain is now on the lookout for an opportunity to binge and it will take it whether you like it or not.

You have less energy as your metabolism has been slowed in order to preserve fat. You have less muscle as your body has been making glucose out of it in order to keep your brain hyper-vigilant. When the opportunity to binge arises, biology will take over and your rational brain will tell you that you have failed. You will give up your diet. With your reduced muscle and metabolism you will end up with more body fat than before and also be unhappier because of your disappointment at your perceived lack of willpower.

Fixing your diet could be an important step towards regaining control and moving into thrive mode. Here is where we need to buck conventional thinking. I want you to eat more but of the right things. We have become too smart, we think that if we eat less and move more then we will lose weight. Our disappointment when this doesn't happen is a natural result of us not being smart enough to outsmart biology. Consideration of how we have evolved to function is at the heart of any long-term physical change.

The following pages will outline what I want you to eat and how much in order to kick start your move back into thrive mode.

If any of the lifestyle factors mentioned resonated with you, it might be a good time to visit them and tackle them head on. The chances are they are more important to your overall health and transformation.

The following is a list of nutritional stressors that need addressing before anything else. These issues must all be addressed in order for your body to reach thrive mode.

1.   Low Vitamin D levels

This is so important to health that your body cannot properly maintain health when levels are low. Vitamin D is a steroid hormone that puts our bodies into overdrive. If we have adequate blood levels we have more energy, the bad things that we eat matter less, allergies and aliments go away and we simply function on a higher level. Fat burning, muscle gain and all athletic performance will also receive a massive boost. It is one for the main missing links in modern health - and it's free!

Vitamin D is vital for: proper auto-immune function (vitamin D can literally clear up the worst case of eczema in a few days), cancer prevention, fat metabolism (very important if you want to lose weight), fertility, insulin resistance (again vital for weight loss goals), type 1 and 2 diabetes, and cardiovascular disease.

I would recommend downloading an app to measure your vitamin D levels while getting as much exposure as possible during the summer (without getting burnt!) the best time is 11:00-15:00, so your lunch hour should be taken outside - without sunscreen!

In the winter, a brief weekly sunbed would be ideal. Failing that, try supplementing with 5,000 iu per day. Consult your Doctor before engaging in any supplement protocol.

2.   Low Omega 3 fats

Omega 3 fatty acids are vital for their anti-inflammatory effect, helping to counter the inflammatory effect of modern life and the modern diet. DHA is the most commonly known fatty acid, due to its role in foetal brain development and safe baby delivery as well as its role in every day brain function. EPA also has anti-inflammatory effects and helps to thin the blood.

Reducing inflammation is hugely important for helping the body return to thrive mode. If you are overweight this is a sign of systemic inflammation and fish oils will be of great benefit to you. Try supplementing with 1000mg of EPA and DHA (total combined) per day. Also, look to reduce your Omega 6 intake, especially from processed foods.

3. Low Magnesium levels

Magnesium is vital for energy production and involved in almost every reaction in the body from nerve transmission to muscle contraction. Low magnesium levels are thought to manifest as carbohydrate craving.

Magnesium deficiency is thought play a role in cardiovascular disease, insulin resistance (important for fat loss), high blood pressure and chronic fatigue. Our bodies require somewhere between 1000-2000mg per day with the best source being dark green vegetables, nuts and dark chocolate. It is possible to reach this with a good serving of veg at every meal and some nuts. Supplementing with magnesium citrate would help you reach the upper range.

If taken just before bed it can greatly increase the quality of your sleep. An overdose will have a laxative effect.

4. Nutrient deficiencies

You are no doubt aware that our bodies are an intricate system with millions of processes occurring at any one time. These chemical reactions involved many nutrients that our bodies are able to produce themselves but, many of these nutrients must be eaten. Our goal is to return the body to thrive mode; in order to achieve this we must deliver the nutrients it requires to thrive.

This is best achieved by eating good quality protein sources and a lot of vegetables. If you are not including vegetables at every meal you are reducing your body's ability to move into thrive mode.

5. Food intolerance

The early part of your nutrition plan asks you to eliminate a number of foods: grains, legumes, nuts, dairy, fruit, processed foods and sugar. I don't like the word 'detox' but the removal of these foods in the short term will allow you to isolate whether your body has been fighting allergies or struggling to digest food it doesn't recognise. This can cause your body much stress and leave it stuck in survival mode.

It's also worth noting that digestive issues will cause the body additional stress but they may well be resolved by the above interventions. You will learn more about this process during the digestion section.

Include protein at every meal

Protein is one of three macronutrients along with fat and carbohydrates. Carbohydrates tend to get the bulk of the attention as vegetables and fruit carry vitamins and minerals. Protein has been adopted by the muscle building crew.

Carbs are marketed for health whereas protein is marketed for bulk. Despite there being cultures the world over surviving almost exclusively on protein whereas others have very little, there are no cultures that have significantly more muscle mass than any other.

An increase in protein intake does not result in more muscle mass. Also, our bodies can much easier support life without carbohydrates than it could without protein.

During digestion protein is broken down into amino acids. Amino Acids are the building blocks of all proteins in the body. These amino acids are absorbed through the gastrointestinal tract into the bloodstream for building and repairing muscles, organs, blood proteins and to be involved in metabolic pathways.

There are 22 amino acids most of which the body produces internally. There are eight essential amino acids which means there are eight that your body requires through sufficient amounts of food.

Amino acids are involved in: hair, nail and muscle growth, muscle repair, muscle contraction, hormone secretion, digestion, water regulation, immune support, nutrient transport, oxygen transport and blood clotting.

When considering health and body composition it is important that protein be the first thing on your plate. As well as being essential for health, it also takes much longer to digest than carbohydrate, for which the process of digestion begins in the mouth with saliva.

Protein will keep you fuller for longer, help to reduce the quantity of food you require and the regularity with which you feel the need to eat. It's important that you feel satiated between meals because it is easy to get into the habit of grazing all day. If you find you are snacking or grazing it is a sign that you are not eating enough at meal times.

A large daily intake of protein is the most effective way to drop body fat and maintain muscle mass, thus maintaining your metabolic rate.

There are numerous questions surrounding protein and its importance especially, from those who train regularly. Not getting enough protein can be the difference between gaining muscle and not. Contrary to popular belief, eating too much can cause weight gain an d is not just dispensed as waste.

Protein has always been associated with muscle gain which often leaves men eating as much as possible in an effort to gain muscle and women avoiding it as much as possible to prevent muscle gain. As a personal trainer of 10 years, I have helped many people reach their muscle gain or fat loss goals, it may well surprise you to hear that when it comes to fat loss in women I more am regularly confronted with those who eat too little food rather than too much.

All dieting cues are taken from popular beliefs and those beliefs are being turned over faster than ever. With all of the confusion, most people will turn to someone who has the physique that they wish to have for their dieting strategy. Those who get the best results from their training will tell us how they managed to achieve their results so quickly. Unfortunately, this type of feedback is anything but scientific. It is unlikely that these individuals recorded the variables in their training and even more unlikely that the only variable was protein intake. Most cover models are genetically suited to rapid muscle gain and low body fat. They are no doubt also following a specific diet, supplement routine and training plan. We are left with is a case of 'after it therefore because of it'. We have an entire industry based on following this system! Luckily, there is a great deal of research available on the subject of protein intake, which is very helpful in dispelling many of the myths around protein and muscle gain.

How much should I eat?

Research into quantity of protein required to support muscle growth and repair comes back with a fairly wide range of 0.8-3.0g of protein per kg of lean body mass (approximate weight, excluding fat). The lower end of this range is fine for someone who is not weight training, but those training on a regular basis have a greater muscle breakdown and require much more for muscle growth and repair. Wild fish, grass-fed meat and eggs are the best sources of protein and I recommend aiming for something like 2-3g per kg of body weight, leaning towards the higher end if you are looking to lose fat or build muscle. Personally, I would aim for the top figure to be on the safe side. Protein can also have the added bonus of making you feel fuller for longer, therefore consuming fewer calories overall.

How often should I eat protein?

A prevailing myth is that the body requires a constant supply of protein as it can only ingest 20-30g of protein in one sitting. This myth has led the supplement industry to put approximately 20g of protein in each serving of protein powder.

One experiment worth noting took a group of elderly men (70+) and took them through a 12-week course of weightlifting during which they ingested their daily requirement of protein in just one meal per day. The result was an average muscle gain of 5lbs.

It seems that it does not matter when you take on your protein requirement, it only matters that you consume enough. Your body is also very adaptable, so, if your protein intake is particularly high, your body will adapt to this. If you are not burning off excess calories, it will adapt by adding more body fat. However, due to the massive satiating properties of protein, it is very difficult to over-consume.

The body is also able to convert protein into glucose for fuel using a process called gluconeogenesis. Although this is not the body's preferred fuel, it does highlight how the body survives when carbohydrates are not available.

It's worth noting that it takes the body around five hours to digest a meal consisting of 40g protein, 75g carbohydrate and 20g fat. With this in mind, if you were to aim to eat the recommended daily intake of protein you would be better off trying to get in two or three meals. Eating more frequently is just putting one meal on top of the last.

I want to drop fat not gain muscle, so why do I need a lot of protein?

If fat loss is your goal, then aim for 2-3g of protein per kg of body weight. It will ensure the best recovery from your training while also keeping you much fuller for longer thus reducing your overall calorie intake.

When you are in a caloric deficit, your body still requires energy and sugars for brain function. The reason we force a caloric deficit is to encourage the body to use stored fat for energy, thus reducing body fat. However, during a caloric deficit the brain also requires glucose for fuel and this is created by breaking down muscle protein via gluconeogenesis.

A reduction in muscle protein causes a reduction in metabolic rate and will eventually reduce the speed of fat loss down to nothing. By keeping protein intake high while dieting, we are able to negate these effects. High protein intake will help repair muscle tissue, while providing protein to convert to glucose.

What kind of muscle growth can I expect?

Most experiments are conducted on individuals who have never lifted weights before and programmes range in quality significantly. Those new to lifting will see more rapid results than those who have been training for some time. Most research experiments are conducted over a 12-week period. During this time athletes see an average of 5-8lbs of muscle gain.

Bodybuilders however will be happy with growth of 10lb of muscle a year. If you are not training three or four times a week, and you are not doing big compound lifts, then you are a beginner.

Protein powders: are they necessary?

Protein powders are probably not necessary but they are very convenient. An 80kg man looking to gain muscle should be aiming for about 200g of protein in a day. This would require three large meat/fish/egg meals. A protein supplement can take the pressure off the size of meals required. Also with busy work/family schedules, lunch can easily be missed and a protein powder can provide an easy replacement.

What other supplements work for muscle gain?

There is only one that has ever been proven to increase muscle growth during human clinical trials: creatine monohydrate.

While there are many others that aid recovery or boost performance but results in clinical trials are sketchy at best. Caffeine is perhaps the only proven pre-workout supplement.

Conclusion

I would recommend that you try and get your proteins from quality sources such as game, grass-fed meat and wild fish. These recommendations are designed to support muscle gain and fat loss for someone who is training using compound lifts such as squats, deadlifts and bench press, and training three to four times a week.

If you are looking to support cardiovascular exercise I would suggest aiming for 1.5-2g/kg of bodyweight and to aim for 1g/kg if you are sedentary.

Be a food snob

This might not be the most foolproof of methods but it is a good starting place. We all have principles that define the way we interact with the world, from what newspapers we read to the way we choose to raise our children. These principles make up the code by which we live. They are like a series of decisions we have already made that come together to make up both the way we see ourselves and the way we wish to be seen by others. There are of course positives and negatives to be taken from this but none of them change the fact that we have them. Often these principles aren't actually created by us; they are maybe the law or they are the accepted norm of our community.

We all come with our pre-held beliefs about food and these beliefs can either help us or hinder us. Seeing food as a reward is the down-fall of many. Reward for a hard day's work, reward for reaching 3pm, reward for a hard week earning; these things cause us to over-indulge and they are the excuse we give ourselves to allow us to eat something that is not necessarily good for us. There is nothing wrong with eating something that is not good for us, especially if we are consciously doing it for pleasure. When we create a reward system, however, we create a loop that isn't complete until we receive the reward.

The same is then true of 'dieting' or 'healthy eating'. We are often driven to this after prolonged over-indulgence. Instead of creating the most delicious, flavourful dish we can imagine, we either punish ourselves with not eating, not eating enough or allowing the meal to highlight how we feel. Our meal becomes a visual representation of the punishment we believe we deserve.

It is important that we begin to see food for what it is: amazing, delicious, satisfying with thousands of taste combinations and, ultimately, a fuel. In the beginning, the way I propose you do this is to become a food snob. Consume the best quality you can afford and let that become part of your identity, accept no substitute. Life is too short to drink bad wine, drink bad coffee, and eat grain-fed steak.

Cheap produce is the way of business. This is not a recession rant; business will always be about supplying a product as cheaply as possible, whether that's high quality or low quality. To a large extent we, the customer, decide what we want when we go shopping. The market will then compete to supply it whilst gaining the largest possible profit.

For Tesco to win custom from Asda, they must try and source the cheapest carrot, whether that carrot is standard or organic, the lowest price whilst achieving the greatest mark-up, wins. This is true of every product sold on a supermarket level. This is achieved in a number of different ways and the quality of your food suffers to the point where the only characteristic that remains is what it looks like. This sounds sensationalist but, I ask you to indulge me. Go to any supermarket and buy a normal carrot and an organic carrot, then go to your local farm shop and buy a carrot. Wash, then taste: if either of your supermarket carrots taste anywhere near as sweet as your farm bought carrot, I will refund you the cost of this book.

If the aim of supermarkets is to achieve the greatest profit while competing with competitors then how is this done when the cost of everything is going up? There are a few methods used by big businesses to keep giving us the food we desire at a reasonable price.

Reducing time to full growth is something big farms that supply supermarkets have mastered. We know a thing or two about how to make mammals fat, we have been doing it with ourselves pretty successfully for some time now. It's done using two very simple methods:

1. **Reduce satiety; if the animal never feels full, it will keep eating.**

2. **Make their food readily available.**

This doesn't sound too bad - they are going to be killed why not make their lives a big feast? Well, the problem is that although the animal might live for less time before it gets to size, it's going to need to eat a great deal of food to get there.

The most efficient method is to give the animal the cheapest food possible: grains. Unfortunately, all mammals (just like us), do not adapt well to eating large quantities of grains. They get fat and sick quickly. Fortunately, antibiotics are cheap and we can give them to our animals when they get sick.

'You are what you eat' is a true enough statement. When we eat supermarket meat, we will take some goodness from it but we will also take away antibiotics and grains from a highly stressed and unwell animal. It's no wonder we are developing a tolerance to antibiotics when we eat them every day.

Farm fish are now fed on soya bean oil, despite it being proven that individuals who eat this fish experience insulin resistance which is a precursor to type II diabetes and obesity.

Buying in bulk is a great way of ensuring the best possible price. Supermarkets will agree to buy a farm's stock for the next five years at a ridiculously low price per lb. The price won't be good for the farmer but it will ensure an income so it's difficult to pass up. From the farmer's point of view the goal is to pay out as little as possible while keeping as many cattle as possible alive and getting them to slaughter size as quickly as possible, while dancing as close as possible to EU food regulations. This means fewer staff, less care, cheaper food, more antibiotics and a reduced land requirement (exercise might make them thinner and it costs money). However, it also means that our animals have had to put up with an awful lot of travel stress in order to get to our plate.

I understand that you might be wondering why all the care for these animals, they are just animals. Just as the quality of what we eat and the way we live dictate our health, the same is true of all mammals. A poorly treated animal that eats rubbish and takes antibiotics is going to provide poor quality meat.

And it's not just animals that these tricks work for:

Supermarkets want veg and they want it for the best possible price so bulk buying is, from the supermarkets' point of view, the best option. Selling veg, however, is a high-risk strategy when there are thousands of customers per store. They have to be prepared to throw away a huge amount of veg if it doesn't sell before it perishes.

Fortunately there are some tricks. Despite it compromising flavour, fruit and veg will often be picked early and quickly chilled to slow the deterioration process. If you have ever experienced the avocado that would never ripen then you have been a victim of **1-methylcyclopropene**. Although this chemical blocks the release of flavour, it also slows the ripening process significantly and is being used for more and more produce.

Fungicides are commonly used to prevent mould forming on your veg. The result of all this is tasteless veg and, with heavy use of **pesticides** in both organic and normal fruit and veg, there is plenty of negative to take with the positive.

Fruit and veg is not just about goodness, it should also be a taste sensation - what else is there to drive us to eat it? I don't imagine a family of cave people would have sat around a fire with mum pushing the kids to eat their veg. The truth is that high sugar, processed food and smoking all have negative effect on our taste buds. When we are met with extra bland fruit and vegetables it is easy to see why we eat them begrudgingly.

Competition and economies of scale result in a significantly poorer quality of food. This statement becomes even more true, if not borderline scary, when it comes to processed food like bread, cereals, pasta and pastries. We have already learned that shelf life is the main issue with food, prolong the shelf life and you will throw away less which will keep the price down. If the shelf life is infinite, you have a licence to print money.

Gary Taubes discovered during his research into obesity that bizarrely it seemed to be a disease of poverty. Ironically, obese women are pictured carrying around children who are suffering from malnutrition. Obesity has long been associated with too much of the good life but it turns out that it's more about too much food and not enough nutrition.

The cheapest way to feed someone is with grains. Grains can be kept for years, they can be shipped anywhere and easily distributed. What they don't offer, however, is any nutrition at all and they are also not satiating. The adult's body quickly becomes insulin resistant and obese, while the children are unable to derive nutrition from them and become emaciated. To add insult to injury, hunger levels are increased which drives them to eat more, pushing the obesity further.

Meanwhile big food companies, such as Monsanto, are able to approach the government and tell it that they have the power to feed the world, do it cheaply and keep a five-year surplus. The government then subsidises the production of millions of hectares of corn and wheat.

Our taxes now pay for corn and grain to be produced, then we buy grain products which lead to obesity, type 2 diabetes, cancer, cardiovascular disease, auto-immune disease and more. We feed the world's poor by sending them grains that kill them. We also feed ourselves the very same grains; we just dress them up as bread, pasta, cereals and yummy stuff like pastries, cookies and cakes. We will eat crap just as long as it has been polished!

The way to avoid this is to be a food snob. Knowledge of where your food comes from, how it's treated and what it eats is a great place to start. Buying from someone who can tell you what your food has been getting up to before it hits your plate is a great way to ensure not only health but taste.

Remember:
- Fish should be wild.
- Beef should be grass-fed.
- Wild game is probably the best source of meat around.
- Chickens should be free range and from a local farm.
- Pigs should be free range and not fed grains.

When you're looking for the best veg, you want the shortest time from farm to plate without any extreme measures having been taken to make it last longer. Farm shops or local grocers are your best bet.

If you apply a similar rule to wine, coffee, chocolate, etc. you will hopefully end up consuming less, but of a better quality product. Make these choices part of your identity. Give them 30 days and you will struggle to go back to eating supermarket food.

Understanding digestion

Not the most glamorous of subjects but a basic understanding of digestion will help to dispel almost every myth you have heard about nutrition. The myths surrounding digestion run deeper than we realise. Many of them are things that we just take for granted.

- Eat little and often.
- Breakfast like a king, lunch like a queen, dine like a pauper.
- Breakfast is the most important meal of the day.
- Eat healthy snacks through the day to maintain blood sugar.
- Eat regularly to maintain energy.
- Eat complex carbohydrates for slow-release energy.
- Complex carbohydrates will keep you fuller for longer.
- Skipping meals will slow your metabolism.

There are many more but that's a start. Digestion is the mechanical and chemical breakdown of our food. Assuming you have eaten a meal of protein, carbs and fat, the following is an outline of is happening inside you. I will try and share enough information for you to understand what's going on but not so much that you require a double espresso to complete two pages.

As we chew food, amylase in our saliva begins to break down any starch you may be eating. Protein and fat are mechanically broken down and remain chemically unaltered until later in the digestion progress.

As the food reaches the stomach, gastric juices begin the breakdown of protein while no further digestion of carbs or fat occurs. After one to two hours of sloshing around, our meal becomes a big ball of what is called chyme. The chyme then passes through to the small intestine where 95% of the absorption occurs.

Protein is broken down into individual amino acids for the body to use as needed. Carbohydrates, regardless of form, are broken down into either glucose or fructose (sugar). Whether you have eaten a spoonful of sugar or a bowl of wholegrain pasta, it will become glucose before it is utilised. Bile is released by the gall bladder and will begin the breakdown of fat in the small intestine.

Throughout the process of digestion, hormones are released to instruct the body on what to do. Peptide YY is a hormone that is integral in telling our body that it is full. When we eat protein a large amount of peptide YY is released and, likewise, although to a slightly lesser extent, fat. However, very small amounts are released when we consume carbohydrate, which is the reason we are able to eat and eat carbohydrate without feeling full. This should help to provide an insight into how meals should be constructed when we are not performing high intensity activity. Meals high in protein and fat with low-carb veg are perfect for when you are in the office all day.

Digestion is a long process with an average meal of 40g protein, 75g carbohydrate and 20g fat taking over five hours to digest. This highlights a number of our myths. Firstly, even after this relatively small meal, any experience of hunger up to five hours later is not real it may be a request for nutrition. Anything we eat will just be piled up on top of the previous meal.

Your hunger sensations are a trained response or perhaps thirst. The same is true of feeling low on energy. Even someone with 5% body fat has enough energy in fat to last 16 marathons; our body is also capable of making glucose from protein using gluconeogenesis.

Unless you are pre-diabetic or diabetic, you need never worry about blood sugar lows or energy lows from not eating. In fact, studies show that the metabolism actually speeds up during periods of fasting. It is thought that this is evolutionary design. During times of food scarcity our mind becomes more alert in order to aid us in our search for food.

Digestion and utilisation of protein takes a good deal longer than that of fat and carbs. If we consume a large steak and eggs, for example, we could be close to 100g of protein which would take in excess of 10 hours to digest. Not to mention the body is about to keep some protein in temporary reserve for later use.

To have a quick look at the take away messages we learn from digestion:

We don't require regular meals for energy.

- Our bodies will run on fat when we do skip meals which can reduce body fat.

- If we skip meals our minds become clearer and bodies more efficient.

- Missing meals does not slow the metabolism for up to 72 hours.

- Hunger is a request for nutrition not food (more nutrient dense meals are required).

- Eating high protein meals will keep you fuller for longer.

- Eating high carbohydrate dense meals is the best way to ensure you over eat.

- Hunger is a trained psychological response.

Digestive health

A recent study found that babies exposed to germs by way of their dummies have a reduced risk of allergy development. The study showed that children whose parents cleaned their dummy by sucking it had a reduced risk of developing both asthma and eczema.

Our gut flora is given to us during the first year or so of our lives by our mothers through childbirth and breast milk as well as via our environment. This would normally be enough to keep us topped up for life, unless disturbed by poor diet and antibiotics.

Seventy percent of the immune system resides in the gastrointestinal tract and it is reliant upon foreign gut flora to aid the innate immune response. As we become more germ conscious our health begins to pay the price.

For millions of years, we lived in blissful ignorance of germs and we did pretty well out of it. Then, in the later part of the 19th century, it all began to unravel. We learned that when introduced to a host (that's us), microorganisms too small to see can grow and multiply, causing disease.

I won't lie, lives were saved here but a little bit of knowledge is a dangerous thing. We got a little overexcited and didn't consider that perhaps some of these little guys were helping to strengthen the immune response and keep us well.

Gut flora or bacteria is now considered by many to be a forgotten organ. However, gut bacteria is integral in a great number of processes in the body, such as fermenting unused energy substrates, training the immune system, preventing growth of harmful pathogenic bacteria, regulating the development of the gut, producing vitamins, and making hormones which direct the body to store fats. It might then pay for you to boost your bacteria with some fermented food such as sauerkraut or bio yogurt (if you can tolerate dairy) or perhaps even a probiotic.

Fuel for life

Diets are built on methods that result in a caloric deficit; I have said words to this effect countless times in this book. An easy way to do this is to vilify one macronutrient. Some people choose carbohydrates, others choose fat. It is easy to see why. If you remove fat then you often remove taste from a meal and so are less likely to consume a huge number of calories; if you remove carbohydrate you remove the macronutrient it is easiest to over-consume and there you have your calorie deficit.

By now you have worked out your protein requirement for each meal, this protein requirement is based on someone following the resistance workouts in this book two to four times per week. You will also have read how to fuel your workouts and your recovery with carbohydrate. All that now remains is to learn what to eat with your protein at each meal.

Fats

If you don't read the newspaper, you are uniformed, if you do read the newspaper, you are misinformed.

Mark Twain

I'm ordinarily not a fan of quotes but fat has been a victim of so much misinformation and misinterpretation of results that it could take a whole book to convince you of how harmless most of it is. It is blamed for increased body fat, heart attacks and all kinds of other problems. In reality, it is possibly the most innocuous of macronutrients, and great for your health in almost any dose. However, some types of fat are best avoided. Others can be eaten in any quantity.

1. Long chain saturated fats (myristic, palmitic and stearic acid) are found mostly in the milk and meat of cows and sheep. Saturated fat is our body's preferred fat for storage and for energy use. Saturated fat should make up the majority of our fat intake which should be comfortably met by your meat intake. Contrary to popular belief, a metabolically healthy individual should feel free to consume as much saturated fat as he or she chooses.

2. Medium chain Triglycerides (or MCTs, such as lauric Acid) are another type of saturated fat, found in coconut oil, palm oil and human breast milk, so very unlikely to be as bad for you as suggested by some. In fact, there is very little in mothers' milk that isn't awesome. As well as being highly digestible, MCTs have antiviral, antibacterial and antioxidant properties. You can also eat as much of this as you like.

3. Monounsaturated fat (oleic acid) is the cornerstone of the Mediterranean diet and is found mainly in olive oil, avocados, nuts and beef. These should also be eaten freely.

4. Polyunsaturated fat (the essential fats, omega 3 and omega 6). Essential means that our bodies don't make them and that we need them. Modern diets often contain too much omega 6, from heavily processed vegetable oils, such as soybean, cottonseed, corn, safflower, and sunflower. These oils are often the hidden content of restaurant food, salads, oven chips and many processed foods. Omega 6 is found in moderate amounts in meat, particularly dark chicken meat and skin, fruit and vegetables. Assuming dark chicken meat isn't consumed daily, these amounts are easily balanced with a diet high in grass fed beef, wild fish and omega-3 supplementation. Many people blame the current obesity crisis on the over-consumption of omega-6 fats, while also holding it responsible for cardiovascular disease, type-2 diabetes, autoimmune disease and much more.

5. Trans fats. Ironically created 50 years ago as a replacement for the harmless saturated fat, trans fats are without doubt the shortest route one can take to death by food. Trans fats are created when processed oils are introduced to heat. They are common in many processed foods such as biscuits, cakes, pizza, crisps, and pastries. Diets high in trans fats can very quickly lead to heart disease, heart attack, stroke, obesity and cancer.

Fat round up

Despite the reputation that fat has in the western world, there are cultures such as the Inuit people and the Maasai who survive on a diet of 70% and 80% fat respectively from blood, milk and meat. If you are not suffering any sort of metabolic damage, you should feel free to eat the first three fats in any amount you choose.

Carbohydrates

Much like fat, carbohydrate comes in many forms:

1. Highly refined and processed carbohydrate.
2. Fibrous carbohydrate.
3. Starchy carbohydrate.

It's important to know a couple of things that are misunderstood about carbohydrates. Regardless of what form they come in, whole-wheat pasta, broccoli or apples they all become either glucose or fructose before your body can put them to use.

Glucose, like fat, is an energy source. It is primarily for the brain but is also the body's preferred energy source for exercise and recovery. It is important to consume enough glucose to fuel the brain and to exercise, while allowing fat to be our main energy source for day-to-day activities.

Glucose is not the cause of all fat gain, as it is sometimes made out to be. As well as brain function, glucose is required for immune support. It is true that over-consumption of glucose will lead to fat storage but over-consumption of any food will lead to fat storage. The trick is to consume enough to support your lifestyle. Assuming you have a relatively sedentary lifestyle that is predominately office based, you should aim to consume no more than 100g of carbohydrate per day, adding more around exercise if required.

If you follow the carbohydrate list in section 7 should make over-consumption almost impossible.

Fructose comes from mainly from fruit and some vegetables and it has an entirely different effect on the body to glucose. Fructose received a great deal of attention from the health industry when high fructose corn syrup was created as a 'healthy' sugar replacement. High fructose corn syrup is both heavily subsidised by the American Government and blamed by many as the root cause of the US obesity epidemic. Billed originally as a healthy alternative, fructose is ironically dealt with far less well by the body.

Most healthy individuals are fine to consume three to four pieces of fruit in one day, although those with metabolic issues might do better consuming much less. Excess fructose is not absorbed well by the gut and can affect gut flora, promoting bacterial growth. When we consume large doses of fructose, proteins are damaged which affects metabolic function and causes inflammation and metabolic damage.

This is not meant to scare but rather to inform you that breaking down fructose into fructose syrup is no better (and may well be worse than actual sugar). It is best to avoid drinks containing fructose as it becomes easy to consume excess amounts. Eaten in fruit with plenty of fibre, fructose will become an issue only when calories are in excess. Given that you are now avoiding snacking and all meals contain protein and fat, excess fructose consumption seems unlikely.

Fibre

There are two types of fibre: plant fibre and grain fibre.

Grain fibre. This comes from whole grains such as pasta, bread and cereal and is basically toxic. Grains also contain proteins, such as gluten, that cause damage to the gut lining. They also have zero nutritional value. There is literally no benefit to eating them at all.

Plant fibre. This is not digestible, although some of the bacteria in our gut are able to digest it. Fibre is what gives our fruit and veg the bulk that prevents them from being just concentrated sugar. The fibre of a plant is what adds quantity to our plate, a very large amount of broccoli will add a very small amount of sugar. Not only are fibrous carbohydrates very nutrient dense they are great for weight management. Fifty percent of your plate should be filled with fibrous carbohydrate of various colours. Then pre- and post-exercise we add in starchy carbohydrate, if necessary.

Starchy carbohydrate

The human body differs from all other mammals, in that it produces amylase which allows it to break down starch for energy and repair. We should try to consume our starch in the pre- and post-workout window. If you have a lot of body fat to lose you might want to be more conservative here; if you have a relatively low body fat percentage, you can eat much more.

Fuel performance

The title has no doubt conjured up an image of an athlete in your mind and it's perhaps a phrase an athlete would use. It is, however, no less relevant to you. When constructing an athlete's diet we must consider:

- energy for training and competition,
- energy for recovery,
- nutrients for recovery and health,
- fat for nutrient absorption, and
- protein for muscle repair.

There are other things to consider but these are the primary external concerns. If athletes don't get enough protein, carbs and fat then performance and recovery dip and the same is true of all humans.

'Performance' is a term that not relates only to competition but also to immune function, energy levels, sleep quality, brain function and exercise performance. These factors effect all humans equally. An athlete may have his or her income on the line but the rest of us have our health, vitality and happiness on the line.

The other side of the same coin is that excessive consumption of food can lead to fat storage. The over-consumption of processed foods and toxins can force our body into safety mode where it spends its time protecting us from things it considers poisons. This can lead to breakdown in proper function of the body. Hormone signalling becomes confused and, even in a calorie deficit, the body can refuse to drop fat.

Fuelling performance is a positive way of framing your goals. Athletes are free from the stress of detail by pointing everything at performance. Obviously they have stresses but, if performance is good, everything else is good. If performance is bad, things need tweaking.

This removes that day to day battle with foods that don't support your performance. There is no battle; they are not on your radar. There are some people in the office who almost never touch the cakes. They don't have greater willpower, the cake just doesn't enter their story. We all have a constantly evolving story that we tell ourselves.

Athletes tell themselves that their performance matters. Your performance shouldn't matter any less; your performance is your life, too. Change your story to one of ultimate performance and you will become a self-fulfilling prophecy of your own story.

Our story is all too often one of 'I can't haves', because it will make me fat, it makes me tired, it makes me ill. The constant repetition of 'can't' is not something our brains can process very well. All our brains can picture is the word that follows: cake, crisps chocolate, whatever your vice is. The constant repetition of 'can't eat cake' just makes you focus on cake.

If you change your focus to performance cake never even enters your mind. Food becomes performance fuel. Food is not a reward; you are not a dog!

Performance goals

Performance goals aren't always easy to set but this is not a new concept. People regularly set performance goals as their driver for improved health and weight management. For example, a 10k, a half marathon, marathon or certain triathlon distances. These events are often the go-to for busy people, although the training is time-consuming it is also not dependant on other people; you can train whenever you're free. The down sides to cardiovascular goals are many:

- It is time-consuming so when you're busy it often stops completely;
- It amplifies and concretes postural weakness;
- It doesn't support fat-loss goals;
- It reduces muscle; and
- It accelerates ageing.

Performance goals are best when they are something that you couldn't achieve with your current physique. I would suggest looking at your workout and creating time and load goals to begin with. From there you might build towards:

- 100 press ups without rest
- 100 weighted squats
- A good 800m sprint time
- A good 400m sprint time
- 20 Chin ups
- Body weight squat/1.5 x body weight squats

The Absolute Health plan

Proteins – you must have one at every meal

Beef	Chicken	Duck
Bacon	Fowl	Goose
Spare rib	Pork chop or lean pork	Turkey
Veal	Wild Game	Shellfish
Any fish	Eggs	Ham
Whey protein shake	Plain full fat strained yogurt	Coconut milk

Carbohydrates

Aubergine	Squash	Broccoli
Asparagus	Spinach	Greens
Lettuce	Courgette	Brussel Sprouts
Cabbage	Cucumber	Celery
Peppers	Green beans	Kale
Tomato	Cauliflower	Mushroom
Onion- garlic	Artichoke	Pak choi

Fats – use freely

Olive Oil	Almond Oil	Flax Oil
Peanut Oil	Sesame Oil	Avocados
Walnut Oil	Macadamia nut Oil- cooking	Coconut Oil- cooking
Butter- cooking	Ghee- cooking	Meat fat- cooking

How to follow the plan

Drink plenty of water (at least two litres a day).

Important Tips

- Always, as much as possible, eat only the foods that are on your recommended food chart.
- Eat a wide variety of foods.
- Try to eat different foods every day.
- Eat whole, natural foods. Stay away from processed foods. Eat organic when possible.
- Eat protein at every meal and eat a mixture of different proteins (eating sufficient protein at each meal will maximise your energy, trim your waist, and assure peak performance). Never eat carbohydrates alone as a meal or snack.
- Carefully pick your carbohydrates. No bread or refined carb consumption.
- Use fats and oils freely.
- Stay away from alcohol. It stops fat-burning in its tracks.
- Limit caffeine to no more than 1-2 cups per day. This includes, coffee, tea, and diet drinks with caffeine. Also when you drink caffeinated beverages eat protein with them.
- Try to drink only water when thirsty.
- Avoid or minimise sugar as much as you can.
- It may be a good idea to supplement with magnesium citrate, vitamin D and Omega 3 fat.

Eating for performance

The above plan is your base-level food plan. It assumes you are not engaging in strenuous physical activity. Our bodies can create fuel from body fat and from protein so if your goal is fat loss then in the short term following the above plan will facilitate this.

If you are following the above plan for fat loss it will help you to have one or two days a week where you include starchy carbohydrate in your meal. (see chart below).

In the long term we will get more from our sport and training if we properly fuel our performance. Our bodies' preferred source of fuel is carbohydrate and carbohydrate will also help to aid recovery. This does not mean we need add it to every meal.

The trick is to sandwich your activity with carbohydrate rich food. Think fruit or a high carbohydrate meal before activity (this could even mean the night before morning training) and the same after your workout.

Starchy Carbohydrates and fruits

Potatoes	Sweet potatoes	Apples
Parsnips	Yams	Bananas
Turnips	White rice	Pears
Carrots	Brown rice	Pineapple
Beets	Millet	Grape fruit
Manioc	Quinoa	Oranges
Jerusalem artichokes	Berries	Kiwi
Peaches	Lemon and lime	Plums

There are a number of foods that are not on the lists. The reason for this is that people respond differently to them. If you feel good on the above plan, great. The following foods are to be introduced slowly. Three weeks on the above plan should help you to establish a base where you are feeling great; from here we can re-introduce things if we want to and see how we feel.

Nuts

Almonds, Brazil nuts, hazelnuts, macadamia nuts, coconut and chestnuts are all usually fine for most. Remember this is not a snacking plan so include them in your meal.

Dairy

If you suffer from any sort of auto-immune issues then this could cause havoc, introduce slowly and watch for side effects like gas, itchy skin, stomach pain and bloating. If cows' dairy doesn't work for you then you could try goats. Remember to always look for quality local produce. This is particularly important with milk as mass produced milk and dairy is almost unrecognizable to the body.

There is a high likelihood that dairy might disagree with you when taken in large quantities. When we are born our bodies produce an enzyme called lactase. Lactase is used to break down dairy in the body. After the age of four many people stop producing lactase and dairy becomes difficult to break down.

With that said, many people are fine with dairy. Beware; having it in hot drinks during the day is like giving yourself a sugar hit. It will make energy levels difficult to regulate. It would help if you categories all forms of dairy as a food stuff to be consumed with meals and seldom in tea or coffee.

Dairy does seem to have potent muscle building and repairing properties, though, and has a great balance of carbohydrate and protein. Hardly surprising, as in nature we use it to rapidly increase the size of our young.

Sugar

Sugar is a derivate of the sugarcane when reduced to a pure form it gives an unnaturally high dose that cannot be replicated naturally. The sugarcane is on average 3-4m high and is only above 12-16% sugar. As you can imagine you would have to chew your way through a great deal of fibre and leafy goodness to get your sugar hit.

A tea spoon of sugar contains 4.2grams of sugar, a can of coke contains 44 grams of sugar. It is also added to processed foods and ready meals to mask the salty taste and also to play into our evolutionary need for sugar.

With that said, sugar is vilified, somewhat unnecessarily. Sugar (carbohydrate) is your body's preferred energy source taken as part of a whole food is preferred and using it as a fuel or for recovery is recommended.

With that said, sugar in its refined form is not something that your body needs and taken regularly it can create addiction and many health problems. Sugar is best taken infrequently or as part of a fruit or carbohydrate.

Legumes

Black beans, pulses, Borlotti beans, red beans, legumes. These are another food group that can cause issues for people with autoimmune issues. Like with dairy, you should test your response to them. If you find you have no reaction you can add them to your starches list as recovery food. Always remember to soak legumes for 24 hours before consumption, although most tinned varieties come this way.

Grains and Gluten

Grains again fall under the category of auto-immune issues, they also have almost no nutritional value. There is literally zero benefit to eating them other than to give your mouth something to do. For many they cause havoc within the body. I have met nobody to date that doesn't feel significantly better upon removing grains from their diet.

Rice and millet have made the list as they are the least offensive grains and can be a useful starch for recovery. Try not to overdo these grains and do measure how you look, feel and perform after consumption.

Gluten is a protein found in wheat, rye oats and barley. Gluten is potentially problematic for all humans. There are also problematic proteins in corn and rice but they don't seem to affect everyone. Oats also contain problematic proteins which is why they don't make the list of recommended foods. Quinoa is not a grain but also contains its own chemical defence system that can irritate the gut.

Gluten and to a lesser extent the proteins found in other grains don't want to be eaten. In order to fight off their consumers they have a chemical defense system that will irritate the lining of the gut. The proteins will then pass undigested through the gut lining.

Our immune system will then treat the proteins as a foreign invader and launch an all out attach which may or may not manifest itself in external systems such as cold like systems, bloating, IBS. Regular consumption of gluten and other grains can lead to gut damage which can lead to major issues. Firstly the body will struggle to absorb any nutrients. Secondly it can open the door to cancer and autoimmune diseases including rheumatoid arthritis, lupus, multiple sclerosis, infertility, type 1 diabetes and many more. All in all, gluten and grains are best avoided or put on the occasional list. There is no real benefit to them but plenty of potential negatives.

Processed foods

Pastries, ready meals, cakes, all things ready made. Processed food are of course of no nutritional value so no benefit can is to be taken from eating them. As well as this they are laced with salt and sugar as a preservative. Reducing processed food is key to achieving optimum health. I won't spend too much time here as I don't think anyone is disputing this fact.

Week Planner

Example	Mon	Tues	Wed	Thurs	Fri	Sat	Sun
7am wake and drink pint of cold water. take supps							
8am broccoli, peppers and mushroom omelette							
9am walk to work							
10am drink green tea							
11am glass of water							
Noon chicken, spinach salad							
1pm water							
2pm							
3pm							
4pm							
5pm training session							
6pm steak and roasted veg							
7pm							
8pm water							
9pm supps							
10pm bed							

For video demonstrations, coaching and accompanying pdfs and much more register for our exclusive members area over at

fitfor.biz

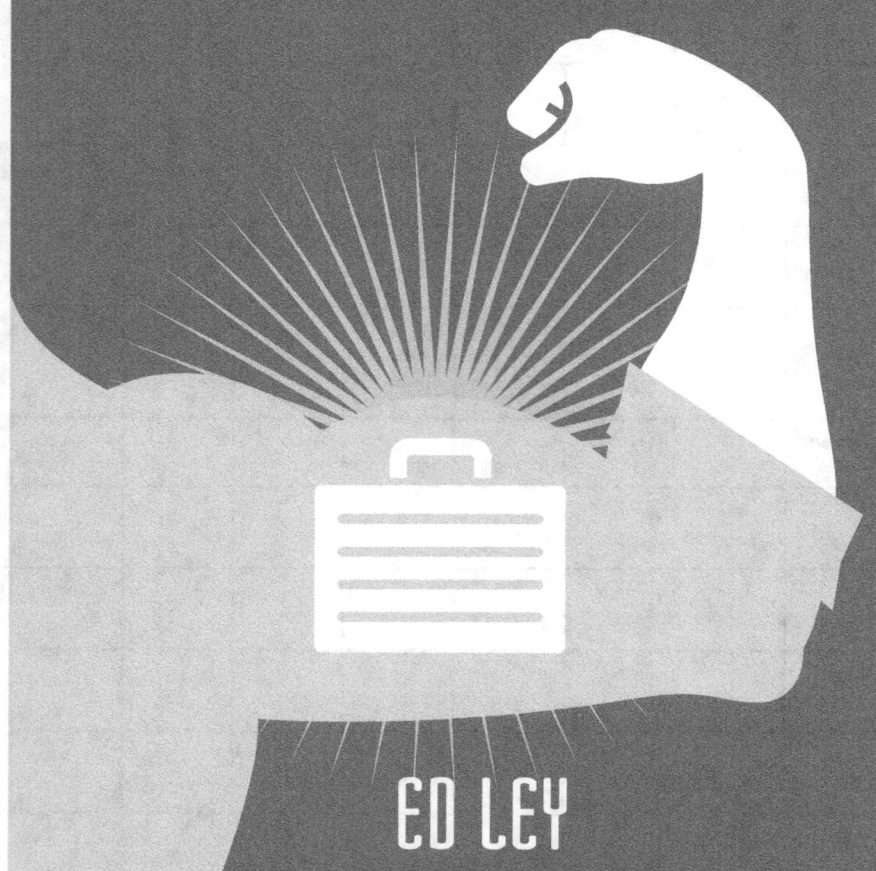

ED LEY

Chapter 5

Move more

A recent study showed that intelligence is actually at its peak when we are on the move. Subjects increased their IQ score by 10 points when they were placed on treadmills, lending weight to the theory that we are literally designed to think on our feet.

From an evolutionary perspective, it would have been the times spent hunting and building that required the greatest amount of intellect. Subsequently, it seems we now function at our most optimal when we are on the move.

When we are not regularly active, both body and mind deteriorate. Although it is true that energy in/energy out plays a large part in weight management, it seems likely that excess body fat is our body's way of preventing the rise of far more sinister health issues. 'Sitting disease' - the new buzzword in health - is one that sort of just creeps up on us. There are immediate symptoms such as increased stress, anxiety, depression and lethargy, but they are incredibly hard to recognise when you're living them. Sitting disease is one where you feel what you perceive as 'normal' until suddenly you don't. Australian researchers recently linked one extra hour per day of television viewing with an 18% increased risk of heart disease (now I'm willing to accept that the quality of Australian television no doubt plays a part here but it is certainly food for thought). It is likely that this extra hour is spent sitting down; you might not place yourself in the 'serial TV viewer' category here and grant yourself exempt. However, for most people, this extra hour of television on top of an eight-hour working day and a 30-60-minute commute. This would indicate that a 10-hour day would put you on par with the 18% increase or beyond, with more work hours or TV viewing.

I could roll out a list of potential diseases and health issues related to inactivity but my list would be out of date by the end of the week. Causal links are made between sedentary lifestyles and health issues every day; it is time to acknowledge the negative health effects and start to create management systems.

Researchers love striking things off their list but, at this stage, they are digging for gold in a gold mine. Almost everything they test is a hit. Science is now showing us what evolution has proven millions of years ago. If we don't keep moving; we're dead pretty quickly.

This is a non-scientific rule of thumb but whenever you have a question or hear a statement of fact regarding health you must ask yourself if it makes sense from an evolutionary perspective. Let the 'experts' argue the semantics of the questions but, if something is occurring that couldn't have occurred five million years ago then it's unlikely to be integral to your health.

Evolution might not provide us with the exact data highlighting what is best for everyone but it does show us where to look. From an evolutionary perspective, we have learned that constant low-level movement, heavy lifting and occasional sprints is how we have evolved to perform. Scientific study has since supported this as the best way to maintain good health and physique.

Trying to implement regular movement into your day is a must for maintaining health and creating a base level of fitness. By using some of the productivity tips and posture tips from later in the book, you will be more able to step away from your desk from time to time.

In the meantime, having meetings on the move and taking phone calls on the move is not only more effective as we highlighted earlier, it can add some much needed activity to your day. Exercise is important but maintaining this base level of activity is vital to your long term-health.

Movement is a skill

When people approach exercise for the first time, after a long absence or even as a high-level athlete, the approach is most often pain in exchange for fitness. In fact, 99% of gym goers seem to make this trade-off. Move faster, do more, go further or lift heavier; with everyone in the gym constantly doing more it's a wonder that physique progression and transformation is so rare. Nutrition plays a very large part in this of course but it's not what I want to talk about here.

I want to tell you why 'work harder' is not a good method for physique and exercise progression. I want to help you to frame exercise in a completely different way, transform the way you train, improve your results and the way you move and feel.

Exercise begins as the restoration of range of movement. Full and pain-free range of movement is where all exercise must begin; without this, muscle imbalances and instability will increase upon the addition of load. When we ignore proper functional movement, strengths become stronger and the gulf between strength and weakness becomes greater. This will leave you open to injury when performing less controlled movement such as sport, gardening or lifting up your children. Pressured or resisted movement creates significant degrees of stress on the body. Stress - whether physical or emotional - can have a very dramatic effect on overall health. Chronic stress is actually the most common cause of almost all illness and chronic disease. Freedom of movement or, non-restricted movement, is a fundamental starting point of both health and exercise.

The exercises in this programme are simple movement of the extremities around a fixed and organised posture (as all movement should be). The movements begin as low-load challenges of the extremities and the core stability. It is through repetition, increased resistance and increased cardiovascular demand that the challenge increases organically, rather than through our desire to push for more.

Once full range and muscle balance has been achieved, exercise becomes the 'practice' of functional movement or movement skill acquisition. The objective is not to thrash your body as hard as you can but, rather to replicate functional movement patterns. The increase in intensity only comes when more repetitions or greater power output or load are required for further progress to be achieved.

A great example of this is gymnastics which is all skill practice but with incredible physique and fitness results. Martial arts can also be included here; movement patterns are learned and, with repetition, they become not only instinctive but more powerful and more stable. Weight-lifting is exactly the same but, mistakenly is not seen as such because people fixate on the load rather than the skill. Skill and timing are required with all lifting exercises - a point that is unfortunately and evidently lost on the average gym-goer. Not that the gym-goer is to blame; after all, knowledge of how to do something correctly is required in order to know if something is being done incorrectly. Replicating an external movement has us believing we are replicating a movement pattern. Controlled movement, however, requires internal feedback more than eternal; the mirror is not your friend.

Increasing the load you lift is not a process that needs to be forced. If your technique is good, increasing a load will just feel like a necessary step. If your technique isn't good then you shouldn't force a greater load, more reps or change your technique with additional 'momentum'. This will all create bad movement patterns that will lead you back to square one and eventually to injury.

Let's take a shoulder press as an example. Our first challenge may be to establish full range of motion: elbows start just below shoulders and press above the head until arms are straight, forearms must remain in line with your ears, buttock muscles and abdominals must be kept tight throughout the movement around a neutral spine (back straight). Once we have achieved this, we select a weight, number of repetitions, number of sets, and a sequence of exercises that surround it (this will affect energy, heart rate, intensity).

If at the end of the workout all repetitions were completed with good technique i.e. full range and solid posture, then the intensity can be increased through load, reps, or sets, or the other exercises can be progressed or changed to alter the intensity of the programme.

Progression has come naturally through neurological adaptation. Your body is adapting so it can maintain homeostasis more easily, should you repeat the act. It literally gets stronger to increase your chances of survival and maintain energy levels.

With a view to exercise over a lifetime, skill is something that can always be progressing whereas strength will diminish with age. Finding a more technical skill to add on top of your strength training will dramatically aid motivation and skill acquisition feedback - you might call it enjoyment.

Performance related goals

Your goal is the foundation of your desire to change so if you get it wrong then change won't happen. This might sound stupid but what motivates most people is usually a symptom rather than a goal. Often when I speak to someone about their goal it will be to stop something. Stop being fat, to stop being skinny, or to stop being tired all the time are all common motivators. The trouble with this is that people don't do nothing - they do the thing they are doing or they do something else. Not being fat is not an actionable step.

The catalyst for action is the symptom: you no longer want to have what you have. The catalyst is only a symptom of why you are not happy. You have told yourself that you will be happier if you no longer have X.

The problem is that no longer having X is not a goal. You need to select something that you want instead of selecting not having what you have. Something that will mean you no longer have to have X. Let's say you no longer want to have excess body fat. Behind the excess body fat is how you feel. Does it create anxiety around how you look? Or your health, your energy levels, your perception of yourself?

What do you want to feel; how do you want to look?

Your goal needs to be something that you cannot have at the same time as your anxieties and symptoms. For example:

1.   I want to look great in a swimsuit on this holiday at this time for this reason.

2.   I want to run 400 metres in 60 seconds and do 20 chin-ups.

Now every action you take in your life and your habits will either move you closer to your goal or further from your goal. It has become something tangible, something you have ownership of, like your symptom before, your goal will become part of who you are. 'I'm John and I lift weights and sprint' is an identity rather than 'I'm John and I'm trying to lose weight.'

If you want help with this process, it's worth looking at Robert Dilts and Todd Epstein's **S.C.O.R.E.** method which can be really useful for creating change and helping you to decide what it is that you really want to achieve:

Symptoms:

- What's not working?
- What do you want to change?

Causes:

- What are the underlying causes?
- What's stopping you from fixing this?
- Who or what is benefiting from not fixing this?

Outcomes:

- What do you want instead of the problem?
- Where do you want to get to?

Resources

- What skills/money/equipment/contacts do you have that will help you to solve your problem?
- Have you faced a problem like this before? How did you solve it?

Effects:

- What will it do for you to attain your goal?
- How will reaching your outcome change things?
- What will you learn from it?

Once you have decided where you would like to go you can then look at what resources you already have to make achieving this goal a reality and what resources you need to bring in from outside.

I realise that this might seem like overkill for finding your workout motivation but it shouldn't take much more than five minutes. Putting effort into the why will pay off in the long run. A proper goal will allow you to create a series of action steps just like business goals. Performance-related goals are easy to visualise and progress is easy to measure workout by workout.

For example, if you want to be able to do 100 squats, then doing 50 this week when last week you did 40 shows a clear progression step. Weight goals are very difficult to correlate to your workout and even more difficult to visualise.

Posture before movement

Although fixing faulty movement patterns is beyond the scope of this book, there are a few tests that are useful for checking the most common issues and will help you avoid them.

Sitting at a desk for long hours takes its toll on posture. Pain is often not an indicator of a new problem, rather it suggests that a problem that you have had for a long time has got progressively worse. According to Dr Kelly Starrett in his 2013 book, *Becoming A Supple Leopard,* 98% of all injuries are pathology based. This means that, after ruling out the 1% of accident-related injuries and 1% of issues people are born with, 98% of all injuries are caused by faulty movement patterns. This makes almost all injuries treatable - and avoidable - when we re-learn these basic movement patterns and they all begin with correct posture. Learning how to stand and sit is a great starting point, and there is only one correct posture: the same posture we use for all activity or inactivity as we see it.

Learning to stand, begin by standing up straight:

- Squeeze buttocks tight (This will level and stabilise the pelvis in a neutral position).
- Drop your arms by your side so your thumbs point forward (not angled across you).
- Point feet forwards and position below hips.
- Make sure ears, shoulders, elbow and hips are in a straight line.
- Engage abs 100% now reduce to 50% (100% could get tiring).
- Pull shoulders back and down without pulling up your chest.
- Tuck in your chin.

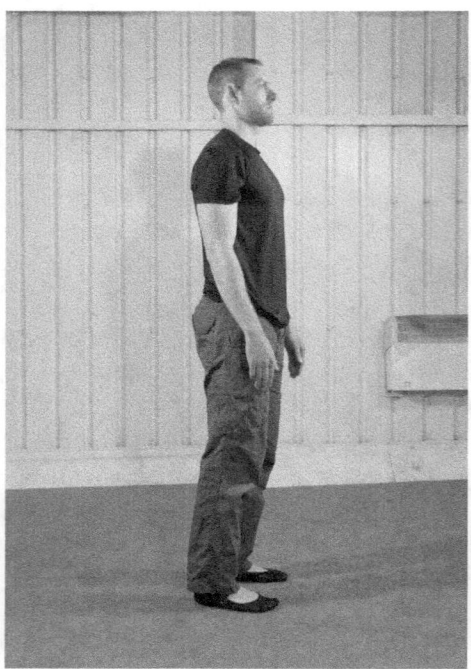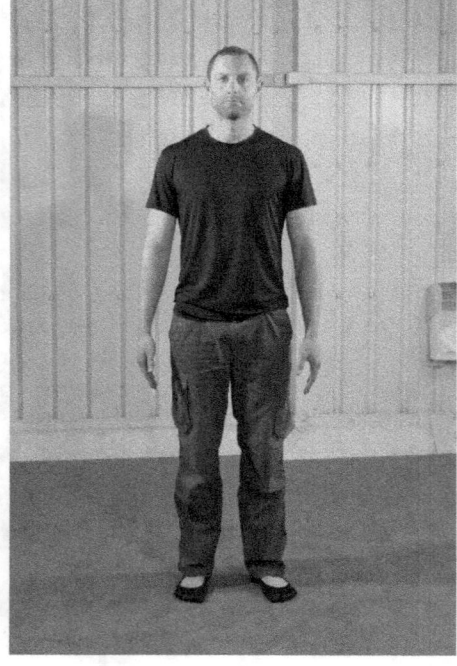

Try to remember the above position as your default position. Create this posture before any movement and before sitting down. When you do sit down your glutes are out of the game due to being held in a stretch.

Maintaining a low-level abdominal contraction at all times while sitting is a great way of avoiding back pain. If you are stuck at your desk all day, getting up every 15 minutes to reset your posture is a good idea.

The best tip I can give with regards to sitting is to do as little as possible. The best sitting posture mimics the best standing posture. Sit tall with your spine straight right up to the top of your head, your abs engaged and shoulders back. Imagine a piece of string attached to the top of your head pulling you upwards.

Otherwise, the message is to keep moving:

- Get up as often as you can.
- Reset your posture regularly.
- Change your seat regularly (gym ball, kneeling chair and normal chair with lumbar support).
- Get a standing desk.
- Split your day with a gym visit.

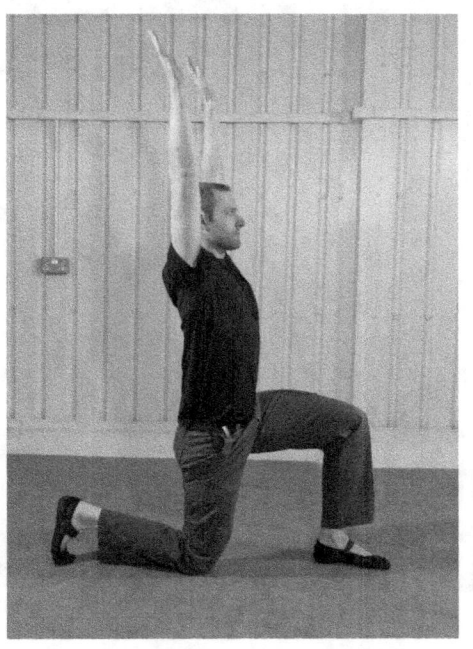

Posture test

Although we are all born with different levels of flexibility, we also all able to move through the same range of movement, give or take a little. Flexibility is more the ability to move through an extended range of movement. We are just looking to regain what you have lost.

In order to ensure strength training is of benefit to you and you are not going to make things worse, here is a simple position that will help to show you where you are now in terms of range of movement:

Your wrist, elbow, shoulder, hip and knee should sit comfortably in a straight line. Without arching the lower back, you should be able to tense your buttock muscle on the kneeling side of your body.

You should be able to hold this position on both sides. If you experience any pain in this position you should seek treatment from a qualified physiotherapist. If you are close to being able to reach the position then regular repetition of the warm-up exercise and perhaps some physiotherapy or sports massage treatment should quickly help to resolve the situation. It is really worth seeking help here in order to get the greatest benefit from this plan.

The ultimate movement tests will be the exercises. Keep weights light until you are happy that you are moving correctly. Never progress onto the next workout until you are happy with the previous one.

Preparing for activity

When we perform a moment of any kind, muscle fibres fire up not only to facilitate the movement but also to stabilise it. The greater the resistance, stability or power required to perform the movement the more muscle fibres are recruited. If we ask for a large degree of muscle recruitment when our body is cold we increase our risk of injury.

The aim of a warm-up is to recruit muscle fibres progressively to the point where they are prepared for near maximal effort without being surprised. Replicating movements that will be required of you during the upcoming activity is the best way to prepare your body and avoid injury.

Warm-up protocol

1. Increase your heart rate and begin aerobic movement (with oxygen). Skipping or fast walking for 5 mins.

2. Star jumps are a good way of moving your joints through a range without muscle resistance. 20 reps.

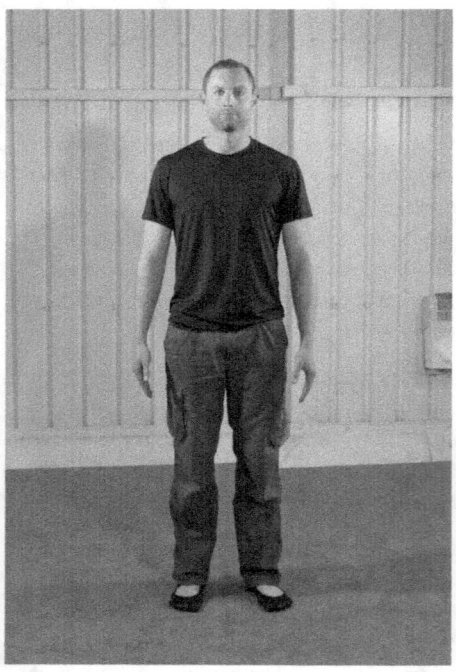 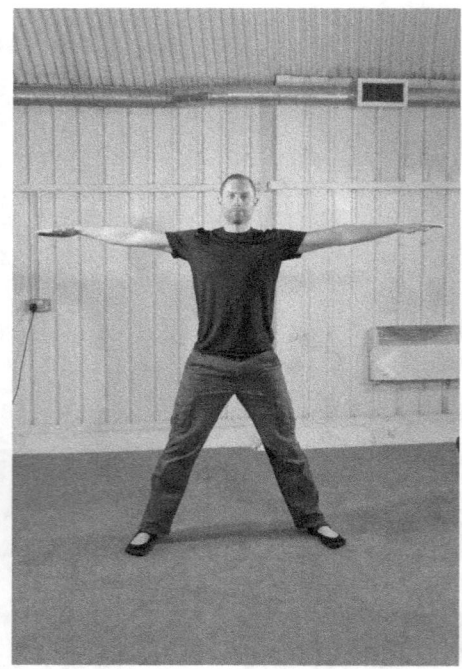

1. Stretches: quad and hip flexor stretch.

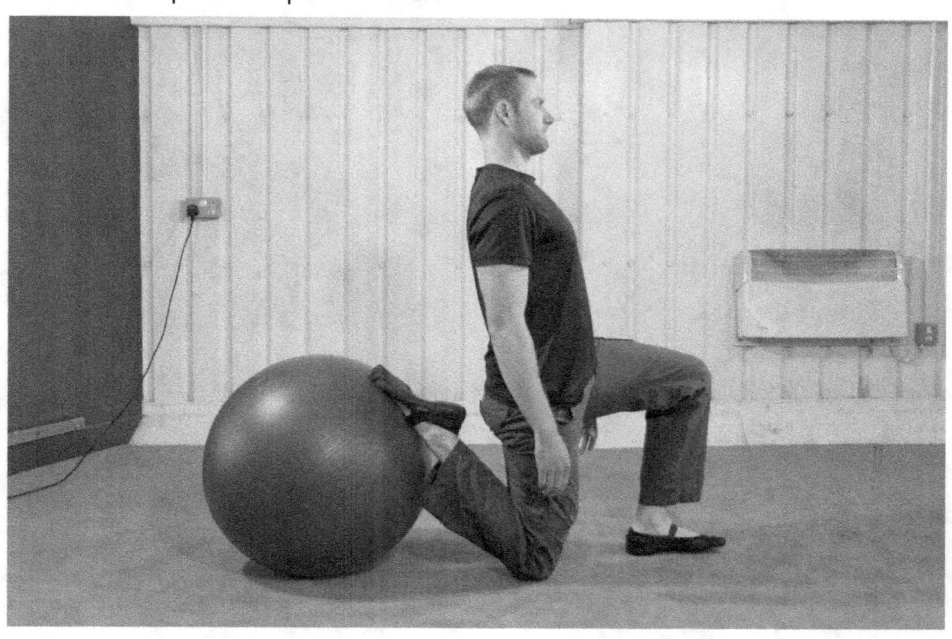

2. Stretches: pec minor stretch.

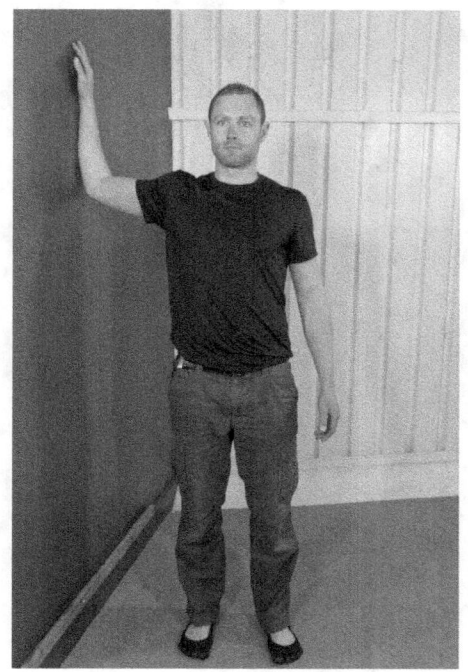

3. Glute and lower back stretch.

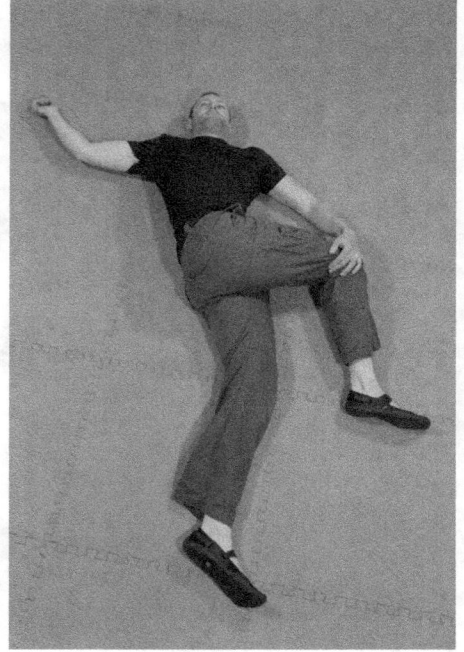

4. Bridges 10 reps.

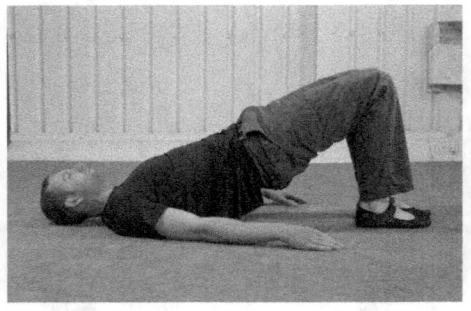 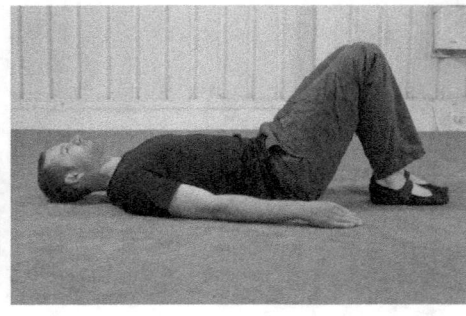

5. High kicks. 20 reps.

6. Heel flicks. 20 reps.

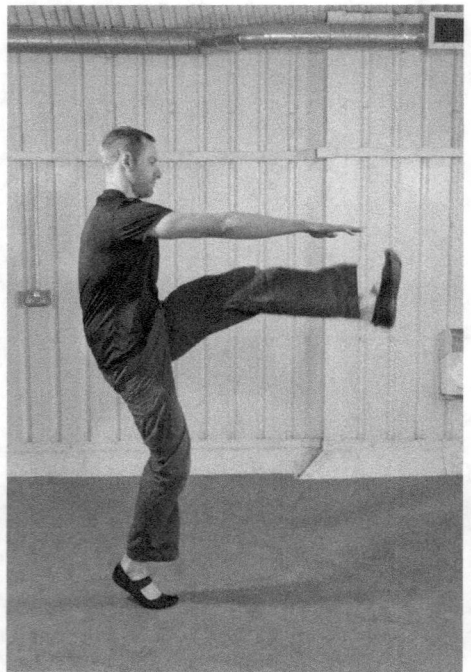 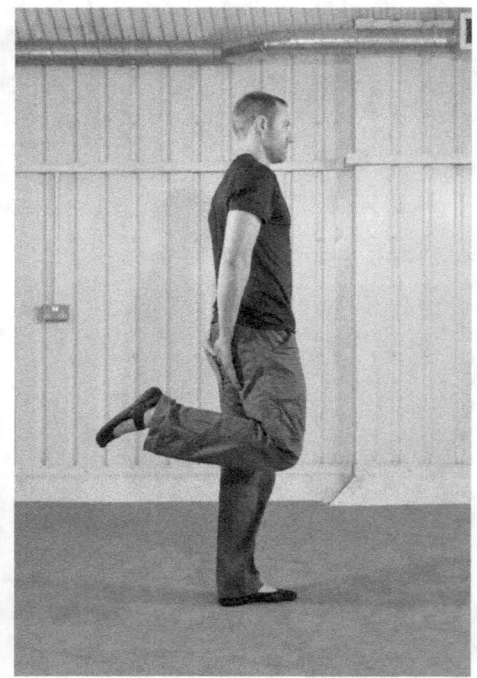

1. Walk-outs. 20 reps.

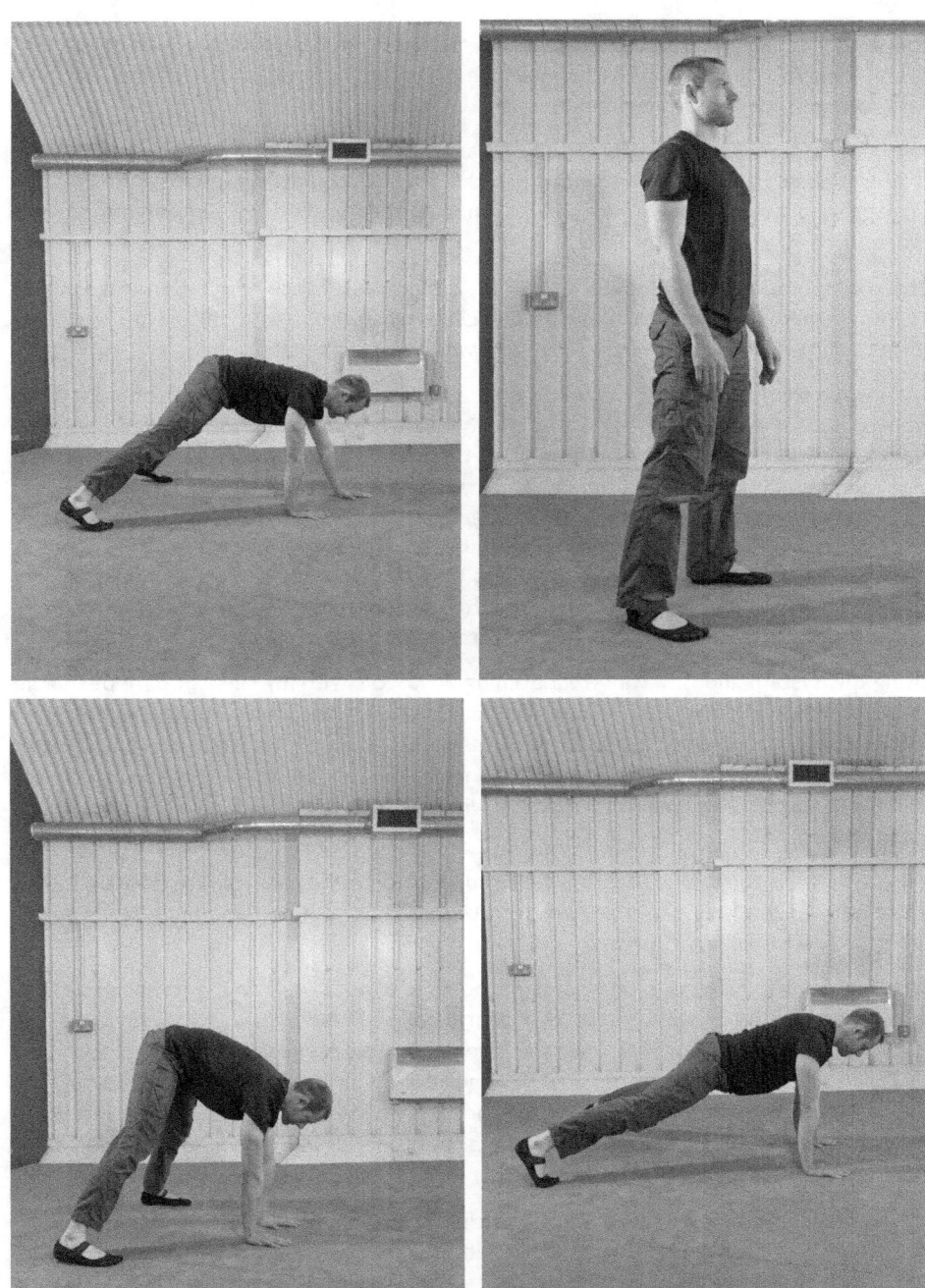

Interval training

You will most likely remember from school days being told that you have an anaerobic energy system (without oxygen) for performing sprints and an aerobic energy system (with oxygen) for performing continuous exercise.

We then assume through observation that anaerobic athletes, such as sprinters, are able to maintain and build muscle through this sort of training. We also assume that through aerobic training, we will have less muscle but a greater level of endurance for sport and heart health.

These observations are relatively true in their extremes. Those who only engage in power activity will increase and maintain muscle, while those who engage in steady state cardiovascular exercise are likely to have less muscle mass.

Numerous studies now show that it is not only possible to have the best of both worlds but it is possible to have better than both worlds. Tabata et al showed that six weeks of moderate intensity exercise (70% capacity) did not improve anaerobic fitness but, improved aerobic fitness 5ml.kg. VO2 max (a measure of cardiovascular fitness) went from from 53 to 58 (Lance Armstrong is believe to be somewhere in the 70s). Those who performed what is now referred to as the Tabata protocol of 20 seconds at maximum capacity and 10 seconds of rest x 8 improved their anaerobic capacity by 28%. They also unexpectedly improved their aerobic capacity by 7ml.kg, improving aerobic capacity at a significantly greater rate than the moderate capacity group.

Using this system and other interval training protocols with my clients I have been able to help them in innumerable ways. I have helped those who are attempting Ironman events and who cannot sustain 20-hour training programmes to drop to 10 hour plans and still come ahead of the competition. I have helped people to burn fat, reduce stress and boost aerobic and anaerobic capacity with just four minutes of exercise per day in some cases.

When it comes to results in exchange for minimal time the four minute Tabata protocol is an invaluable tool and will feature heavily in your programming, along with other interval training protocols.

Those training for physique or fat loss purposes are most likely trying to burn as many calories as possible in a bid to create a caloric deficit. The downside of steady state cardiovascular exercise is that, unless it is completed a very high intensity for over an hour and a half, it seems to create an up regulation in hunger. We burn calories but we also eat enough to counteract any fat burning effects. When we try to outsmart this system by monitoring our food intake our body responds with a down-regulation in energy expenditure, making us more tired.

From an evolutionary perspective, it is possible that our body perceives cardiovascular exercise as us being chased. Two million years ago exercise was not a pastime, it was a side effect of building, fighting, hunting and running for your life. It is possible that the endorphin high that accompanies cardiovascular exercise is our body's reward system designed to encourage us to replicate this running behaviour the next time we are in a life-or-death situation.

This up-regulation in hunger or down-regulation in energy fits perfectly with the idea that our bodies are trying to restore energy levels as quickly as possible in case another hasty retreat is required. Whatever the mechanism at work here, cardiovascular exercise has its benefits but fat burning is not one of them.

Resistance training

Achieving the sort of bulk that you see on a bodybuilder is a full time job. Bodybuilders train for hours at a time and eat up to 10 meals a day. In addition, they are receiving some anabolic assistance.

Gyms all over the world are filled with men lifting weights day in, day out in a quest to pack on muscle, and 99% of them make little or no change in physique. The bodybuilding myth goes deep; it convinces the aspirational that it can be achieved through weightlifting alone, while striking fear into those who fear muscle gain.

Resistance training might well be the single most important change you can make to improve your health and longevity. In 2013, researchers took 48 elderly males (65-75 years old; the study called them elderly, I have some 70-year-old clients that would kick my arse if I called them elderly) and randomly assigned them to one of two groups. One group performed cardiovascular exercise (CV) and the other a mixture of cardio and resistance training. The study was designed to monitor changes in blood pressure and body fat. Exercising three times per week over a nine-month period with no designed dietary changes, both groups experienced a drop in blood pressure. However, the resistance training group experienced a greater drop in resting blood pressure and an average drop of 2.3% body fat.

With three million people in the UK currently suffering from osteoporosis and age (and being female) being a major determining factor in getting it, we are potentially all on a course for getting this disease at some point. Studies have shown that resistance training is the only exercise that proves to increase bone density.

Adults lose on average 1lb of muscle and gain 1lb of fat every year from the age of 30. Our energy levels, ease of movement, mental health, physical health and biological health are all closely linked to our posture and strength. Resistance training will make you look good in your swimsuit but its importance is far more to do with health and longevity than it is aesthetics. Without resistance training, our bodies do not work properly. This is indisputable fact.

Today, healthy eating, good quality of sleep, sun exposure and regular exercise have become choices. The reason for the deterioration of health in the world population is choice. Humans have evolved in a world without technology where manual labour was the only way to be clothed, fed, watered, sheltered and protected.

Resistance training is the easiest way for us to replicate what our bodies are designed to do in order to function properly. You can pay for help to perform both flexibility and resistance training in the form of classes or 1-2-1 assistance. Unfortunately, the seller may try to overcomplicate the process to make it less accessible.

Flexibility and perfect functional movement are things we are born performing perfectly. Any form of exercise designed to improve your life is based around returning to this early perfection. Dependent upon how far away you have moved from what you once had, it can be a difficult process that requires assistance. You are not, however, attempting to achieve something that you have never had.

You were once able to squat, crawl, roll and reach the same as every other human on the planet. Your goal with exercise is to return to this level of functionality and then improve on it. Subsequently, movement is far better for increasing range of movement than static stretching. As a baby, you didn't have a training regime or a coach telling you correct movement patterns, you just moved.

The reason coaching is required as an adult is because the way we live our lives has have made many of these movements difficult to achieve. The aim of this exercise section is to help you return to how you moved as a baby. At this time you had the same movement potential as everyone else on the planet. The closer you can get to returning to this level of functionality, the greater you will perform on every level.

The first phase of this is postural correction. If you had difficultly performing the test in the postural correction section, you might require the help of a good personal trainer or physiotherapist.

If you were able to perform the test, you are ready to start training. Each exercise movement begins by assuming the brace position from the posture section. Each exercise then challenges your ability to maintain this core stability while taking your limbs through a range of movement. Take boxing or golf as an example - the force behind a punch or swing doesn't come from your arms, rather it comes from having a comfortable range of movement and the ability to maintain a stable core and generate torque through it. All exercise is the same as this. With that in mind, exercise should be viewed as a skill. Once you are able to perform a movement the specified number of times with the specified load, you need to advance to a more difficult skill in order to continue to improve.

Improvements are made by increasing intensity of movement, increasing speed, or load, or reducing time taken to complete the same amount of work.

The exercises involved in your programmes are set out below, followed by a series of workouts that should take a maximum of 20 minutes. The function of this book is to derive maximum benefit in minimum time.

Therefore all exercises are all either body weight or require kettlebells only. This will allow you to purchase the equipment and train at home or in a hotel room if you are pressed for time and unable to make it to the gym.

Bodyweight squat

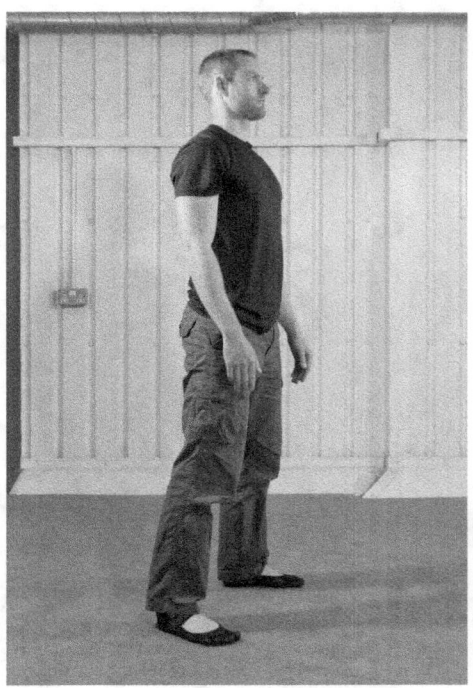 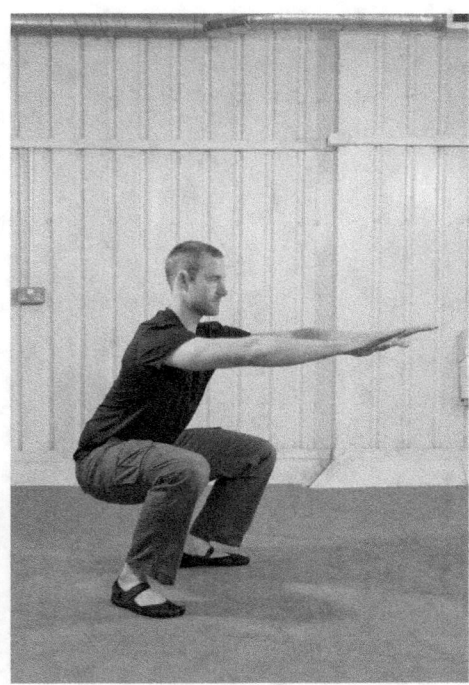

1. Set your posture (shoulders down, head up, glutes tight, abs tight).
2. Stand with your feet slightly wider than shoulder width apart and pointing forwards.
3. Push your hips backwards.
4. Push your knees forwards towards the outside and front of your feet.
5. Keeping your chest high, sit down on an imaginary chair.
6. Go as deep as you can while maintaining a straight back* (in conjunction with your hip stretch this will improve the more you do).
7. Press down through your heels and squeeze your thighs to return to posture set position.
8. Repeat as advised.

*If you struggle with depth try raising your heels with some 1-2kg weight plates

Backward lunge

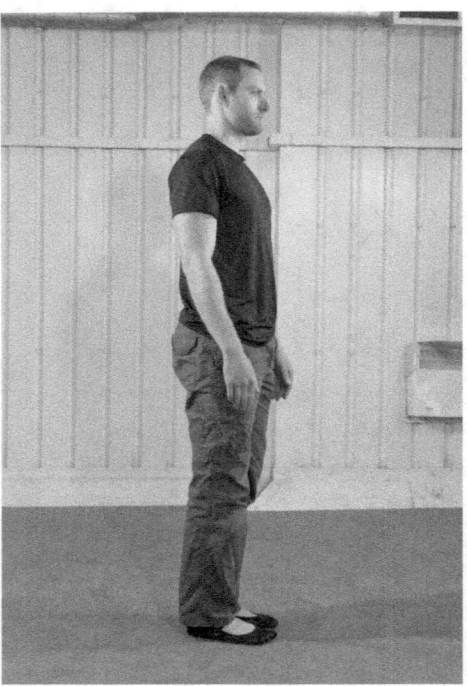 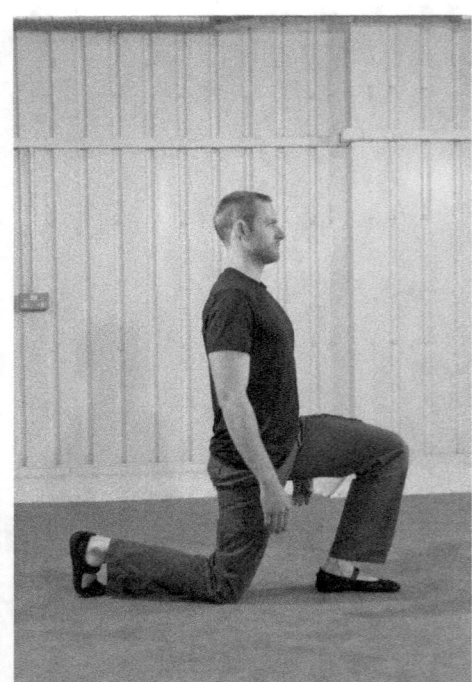

1. Set your posture (shoulders down, head up, glutes tight, abs tight).
2. Raise one leg off the floor and push hips backwards.
3. Stride backwards and place your toe down with leg extended behind you.
4. Loading through the heel of your front foot lower your back knee to the floor.
5. At the bottom of the movement you should still be supporting your weight.
6. Your knee, hip, spine, shoulder and ear should all be in a straight line.
7. Now press down through your front heel and squeeze your hips forward...
8. Return to set posture position.
9. Repeat as directed.

Burpees

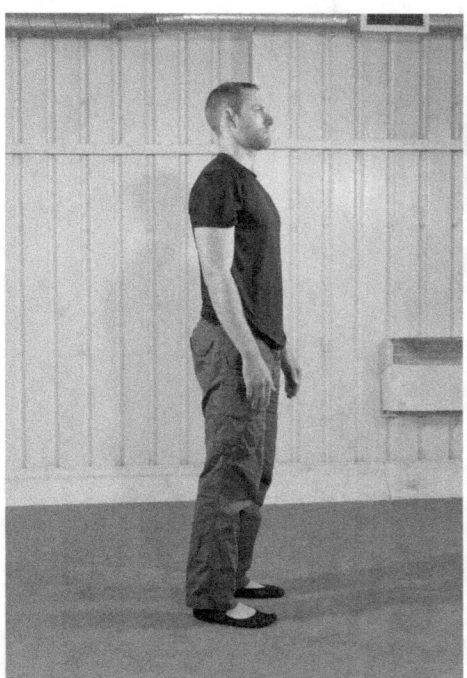

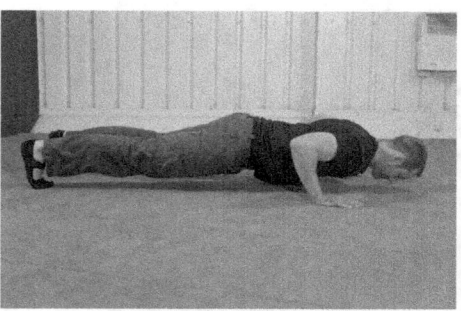

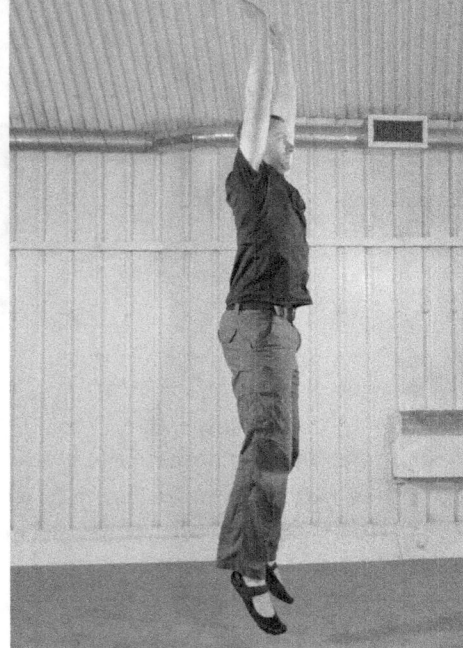

1. Set your posture (shoulders down, head up, glutes, tight abs tight).

2. Bent your knees and place hands down beneath your shoulders.

3. Jump back until your body is fully extend in a press-up position.

4. Lower to the floor.

5. Complete a press up - be sure to avoid arching lower back.

6. Jump forward until your feet are flat on the floor.

7. Transfer your weight onto your feet from your hands.

8. Jump up with arms raised.

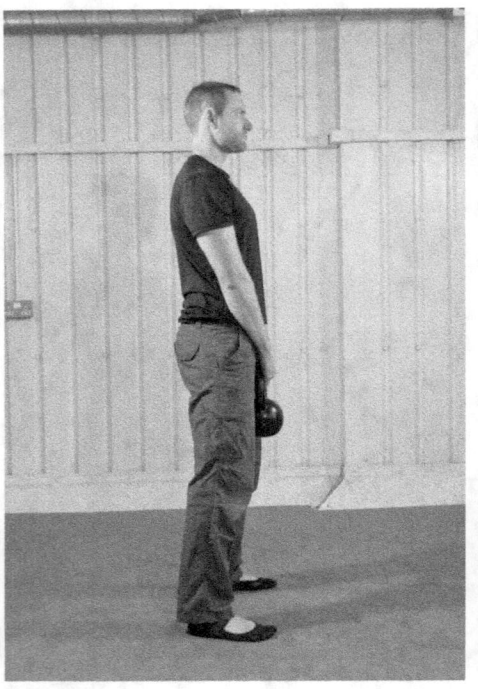
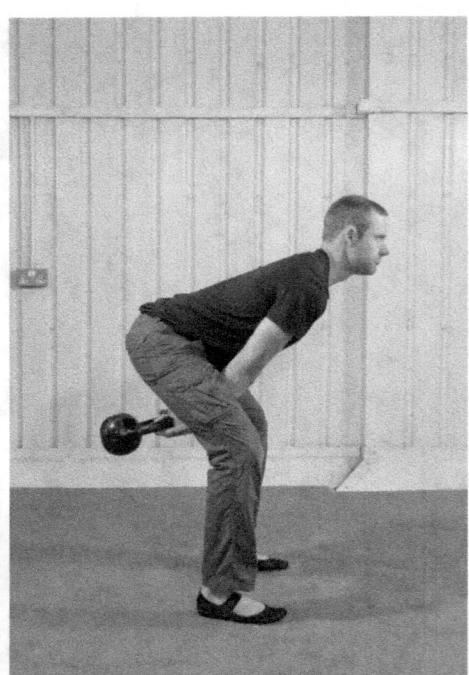

1. Set your posture (shoulders down, head up, glutes tight, abs tight).
2. Push hips backwards and relax your arms, holding kettlebell in both hands.
3. Ensure hips are as far backwards as you can push them and swing kettlebell back.
4. Drive your hips forward as if you are trying to jump forwards.
5. Allow the kettlebell's movement to come from the power in the movement of the hips; it should arc upwards.
6. As the kettlebell reaches the top of the arc, your body should be in set posture position.
7. As kettlebell falls, sit your hips back again.
8. Repeat as directed.

Visit http://absolute-health.co.uk/exercise-demonstrations/ for video demonstration

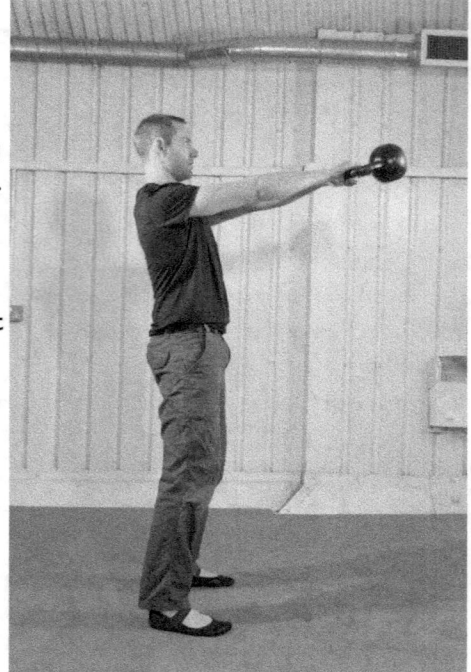

Bench single arm row

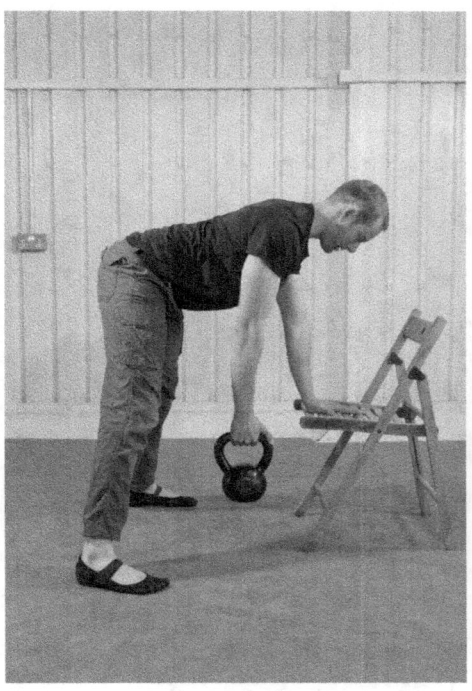 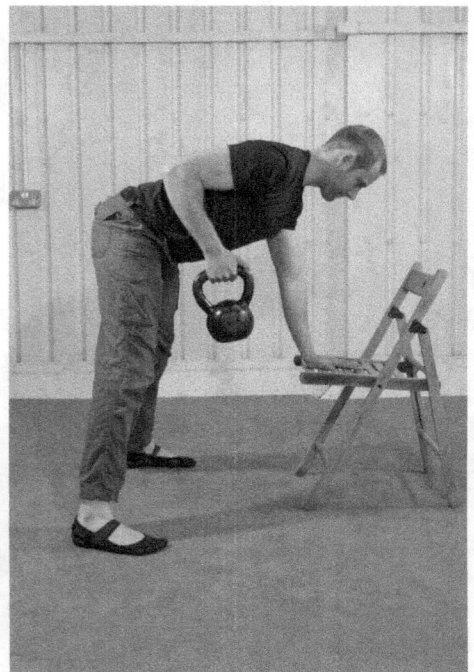

1. Set your posture (shoulder down, head up, glutes tight, abs tight).
2. Push hips backwards to bend forwards, placing one arm on chair.
3. Maintain abdominal and shoulder posture.
4. On weighted side, start with a straight arm.
5. Pull weight up by pulling your elbow towards your hip.
6. Slowly lower the weight back down again, until your arm is completely straight.
7. Repeat as advised.

Bent over row

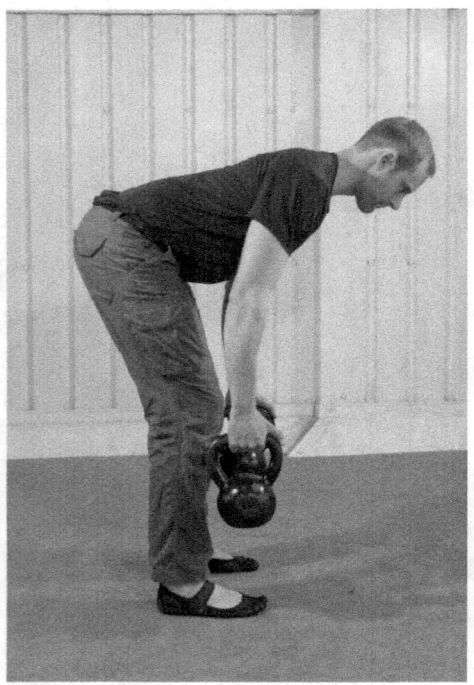 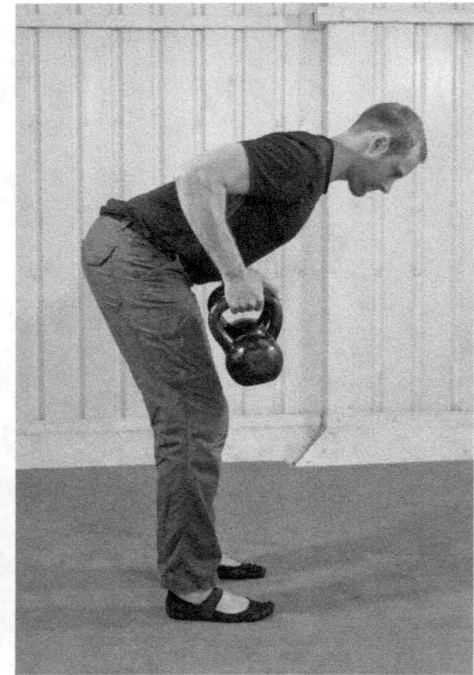

1. Set your posture (shoulders down, head up, glutes tight, abs tight).
2. Push hips backwards to bend forwards (you should feel a hamstring stretch).
3. Reassess all postural queues apart from glutes.
4. Pull weights up pushing elbows towards hips and squeezing shoulder blades together.
5. Keep shoulders squeezed as you lower the weights under control to a straight arm.
6. Repeat as recommended.

Kneeling press-up

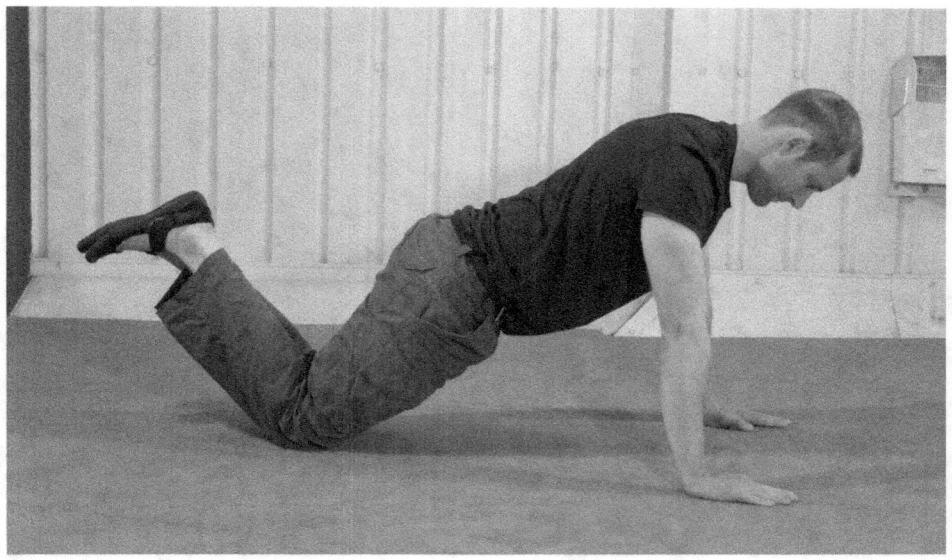

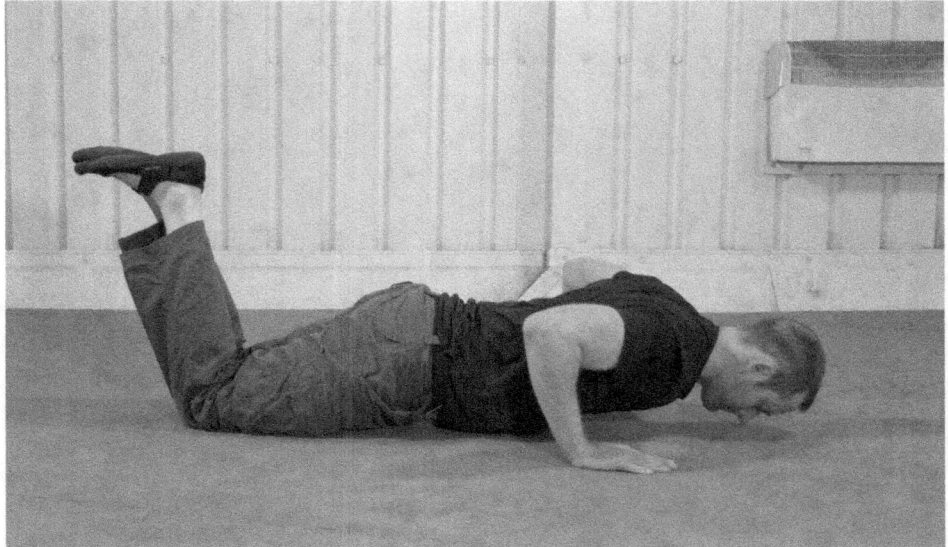

1. Assume the kneeling press-up position and set your posture.
2. Place hands slightly wider than shoulders.
3. Maintaining set posture, lower your body towards the floor.
4. When your nose reaches the floor push up through the heel of your palm.
5. Repeat as recommended.

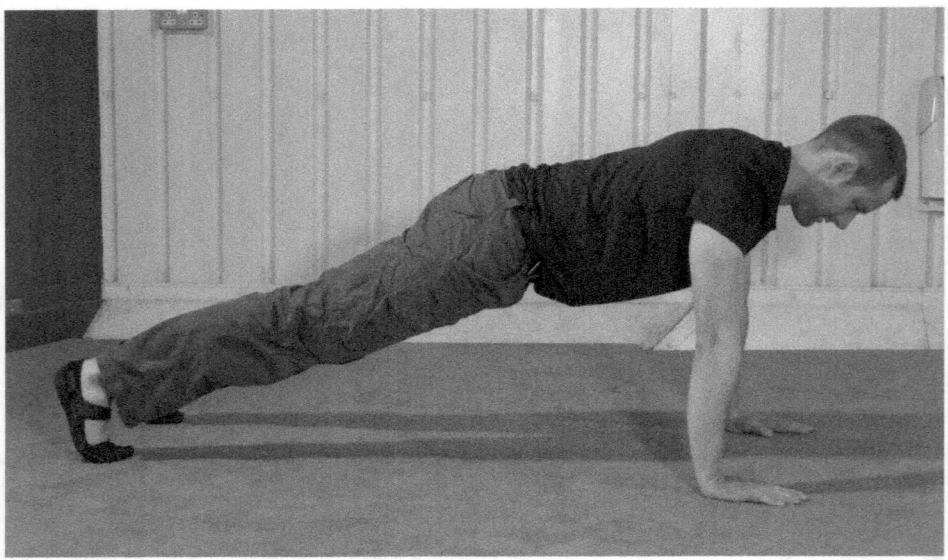

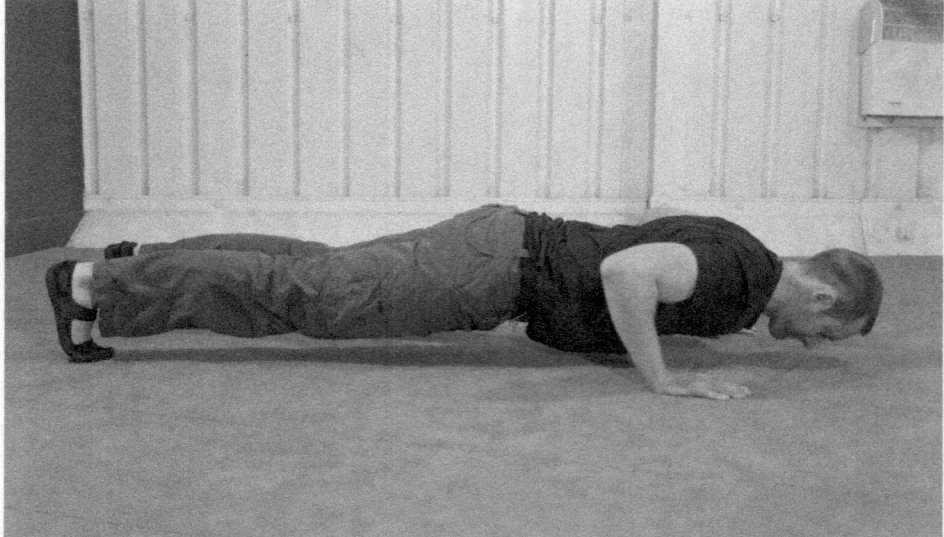

1. Assume the press up position and set your posture.
2. Place hands slightly wider than shoulders.
3. Maintaining set posture lower your body towards the floor.
4. Screw your hands into the floor (trying to rotate hands outwards).
5. When your nose reaches the floor push up through the heel of your palm.
6. Repeat as recommended.

Kettlebell Deadlift

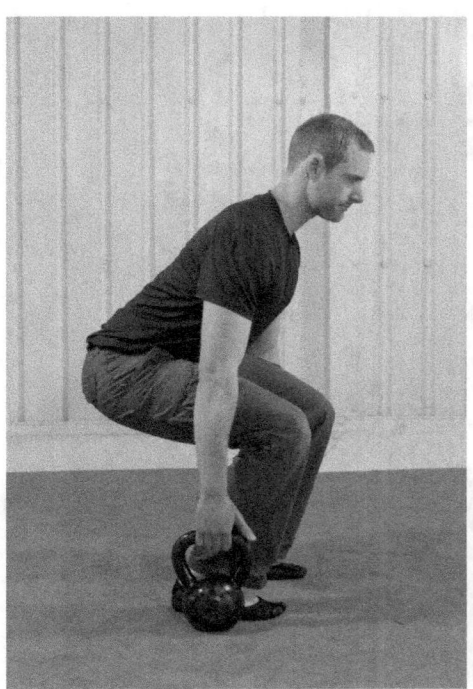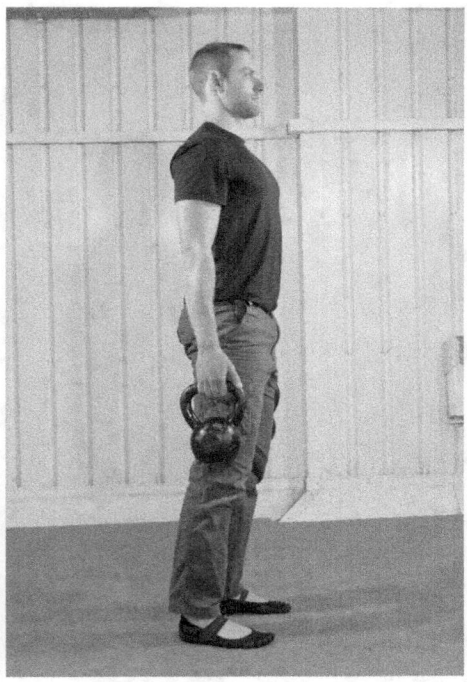

1. Set your posture (shoulder down, head up, glutes tight, abs tight), with weights on the floor next to your ankles
2. Sit your hips backwards until your hands reach the kettlebells.
3. Lift your chest and ensure your back is straight.
4. Lifting weights drive your hips forward returning to set posture.
5. To lower weights sit your hips backwards until kettlebells reach the floor.
6. Repeat movement.

Kettlebell Squat

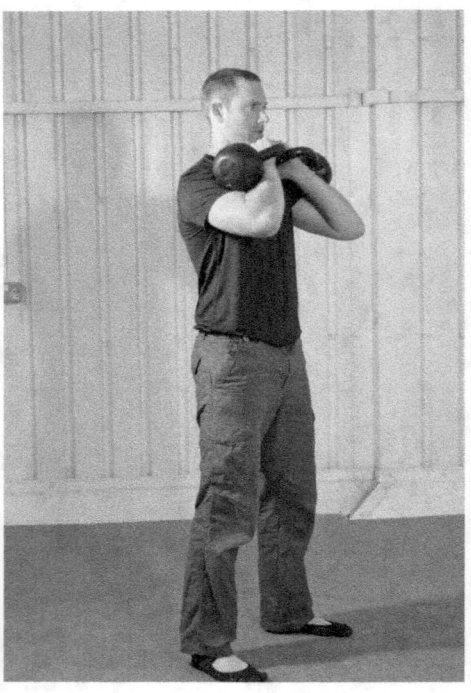 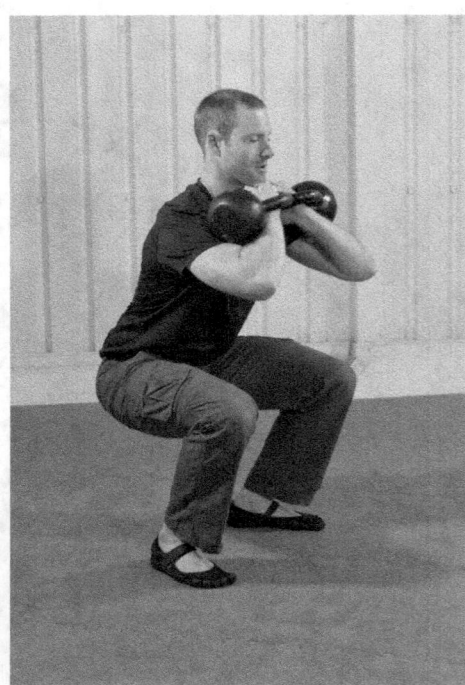

1. Set your posture (shoulders down, head up, glutes tight, abs tight).
2. Raise the kettlebells up to your chest, resting the bells on your biceps.
3. Stand with your feet slightly wider than shoulder width apart and pointing forwards.
4. Push your hips backwards.
5. Push your knees forwards towards the outside and front of your feet.
6. Keeping your chest high, sit down on an imaginary chair.
7. Go as deep as you can while maintaining a straight back* (in conjunction with your hip stretch this will improve the more you do it).
8. Press down through your heels and squeeze your thighs to return to posture set position.
9. Repeat as directed.

*If you struggle with depth try raising your heels with some 1-2kg weight plates

Dead Row

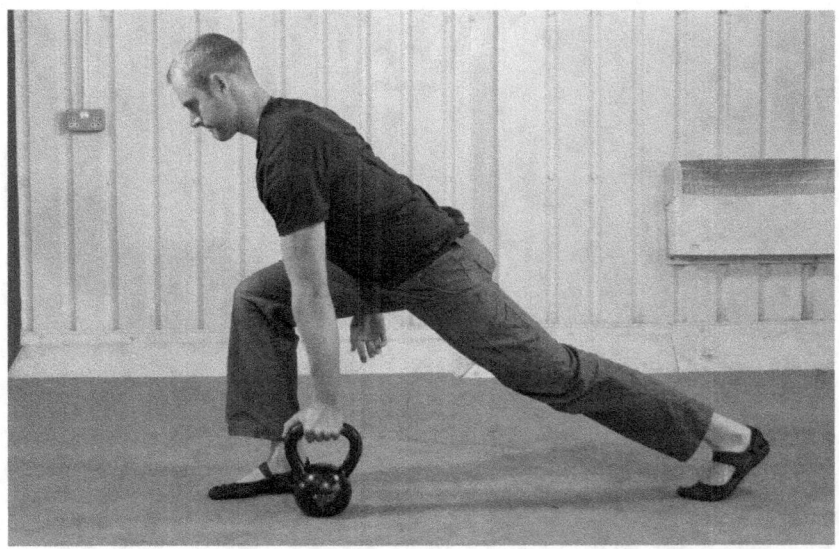

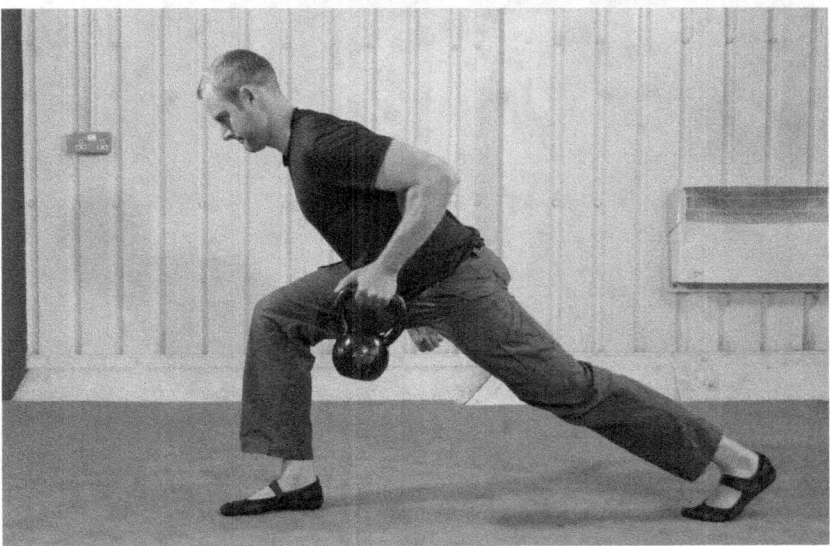

1. Set your posture (shoulders down, head up, glutes tight, abs tight).

2. Place your right foot next to the kettlebell and extend your left leg back.

3. Drop your weight forwards over your front foot until your arm reaches the weight handle.

4. Reassess all postural cues.

5. Pull weights up, pulling elbows towards hips and squeezing shoulder blades together.

6. Keep shoulder blades squeezed as you lower the weights under control back to the floor.

7. Swap your stance to repeat on the other arm.

8. Repeat as advised.

Shoulder press

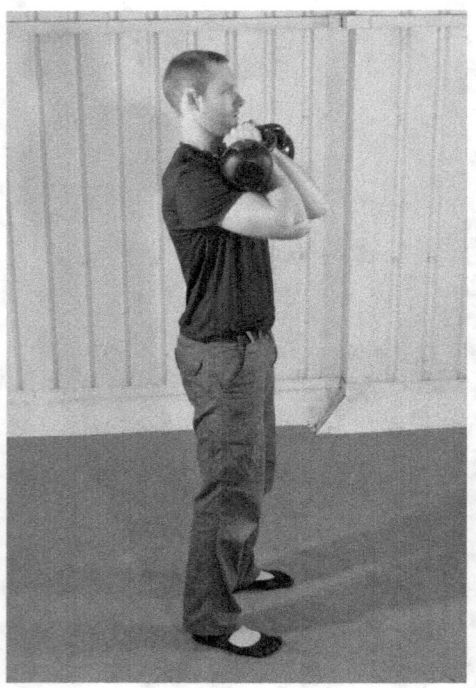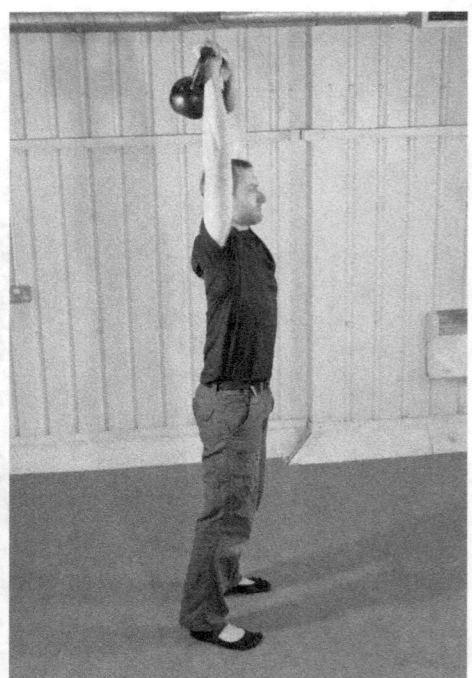

1. Set your posture (shoulders down, head up, glutes tight, abs tight).
2. Raise the kettlebells up to your chest and rest them on your biceps
3. Brace your posture and press the kettlebell above your head.
4. At full extension, your elbows and wrists should be in line with shoulders, spine, hips, knees and ankles.
5. Lower the weights slowly back to your chest.
6. Repeat as recommended.

Push press

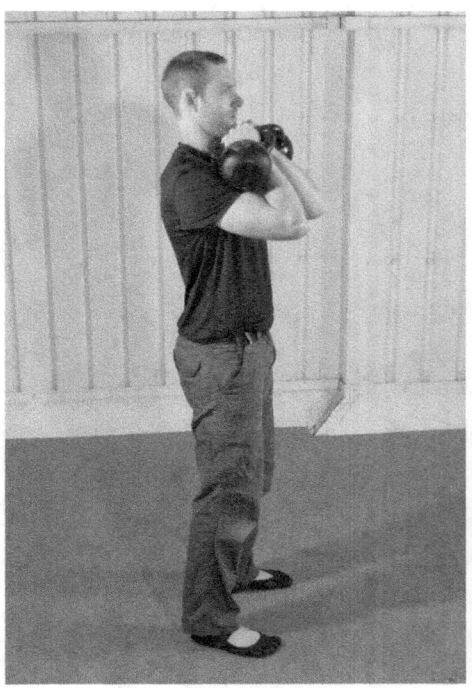
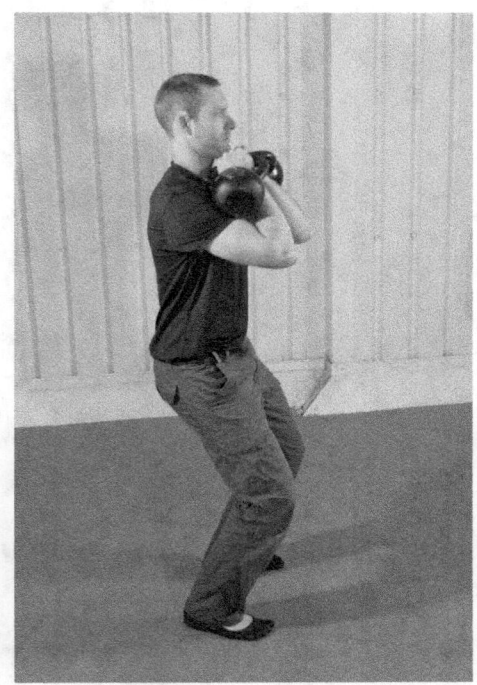
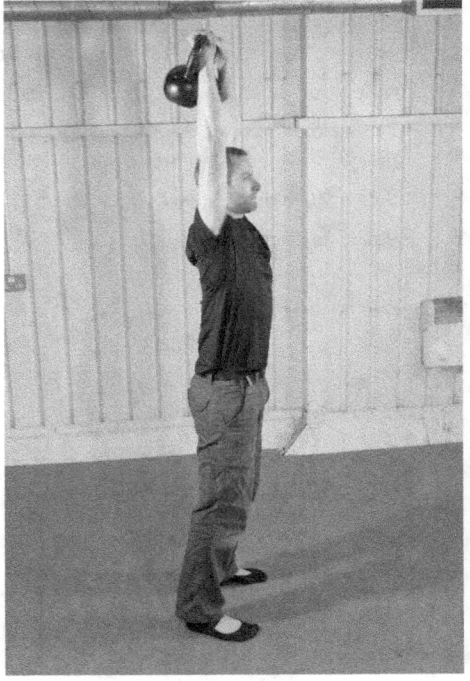

1. Set your posture (shoulders down, head up, glutes tight abs tight).

2. Raise the kettlebells up to your chest and rest the bell on your biceps.

3. Bend your knees slightly forwards maintaining upright posture.

4. Drive body upwards and powerfully press the kettlebell above your head.

5. At full extension, your elbows and wrists should be in line with shoulders, spine, hips, knees and ankles.

6. Lower the weights slowly back to your chest.

7. Repeat as recommended.

Single arm shoulder press

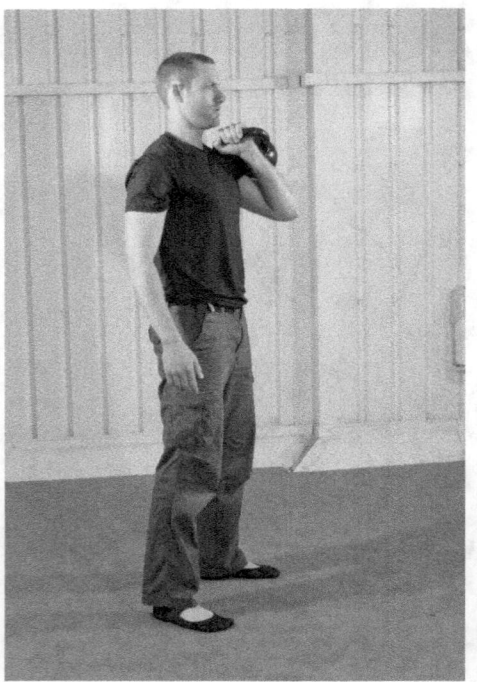 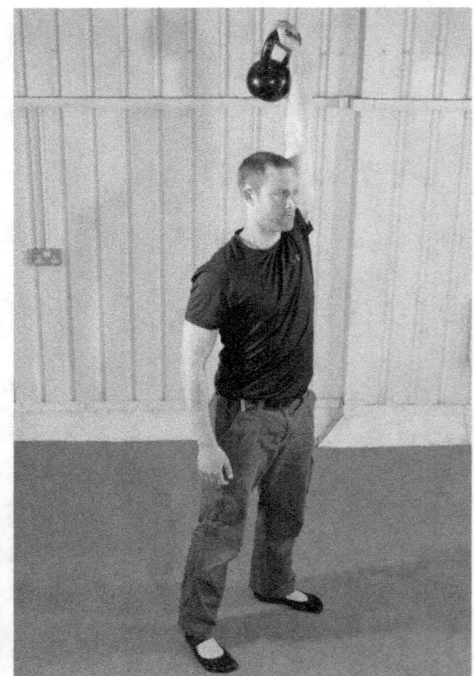

1. Set your posture (shoulders down, head up, glutes tight, abs tight).
2. Raise the kettlebell up to your chest and rest it on your biceps.
3. Brace your posture and press the kettlebell above your head.
4. At full extension, your elbows and wrists should be in line with your shoulders, spine, hips, knees and ankles.
5. Lower the weight slowly back to your chest.
6. Repeat as recommended.

Single arm push press

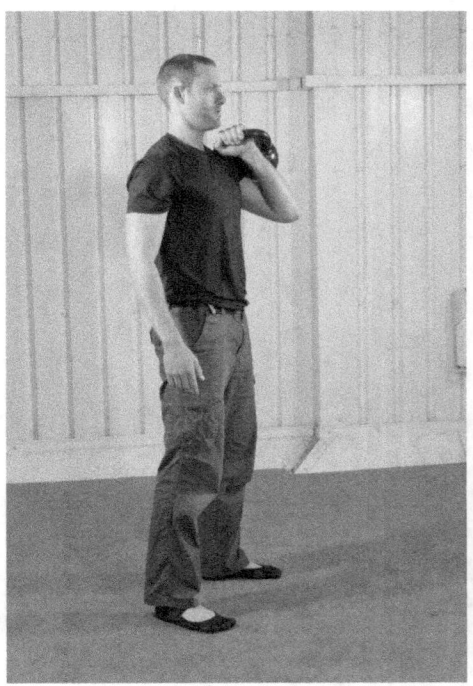
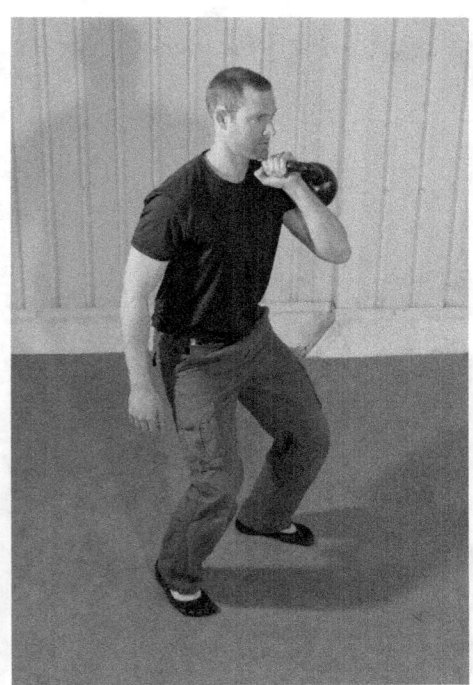

1. Set your posture (shoulders down, head up, glutes tight, abs tight).

2. Raise the kettlebells up to your chest and rest the bell on your biceps.

3. Bend your knees slightly forwards maintaining upright posture.

4. Drive body upwards and powerfully press the kettlebell above your head.

5. At full extension, your elbows and wrists should be in line with your shoulders, spine, hips, knees and ankles.

6. Lower the weight slowly back to your chest.

7. Repeat as recommended.

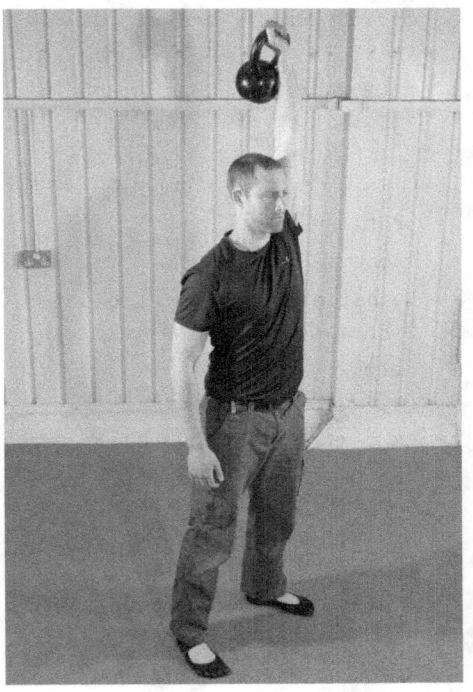

Single arm Squat to press

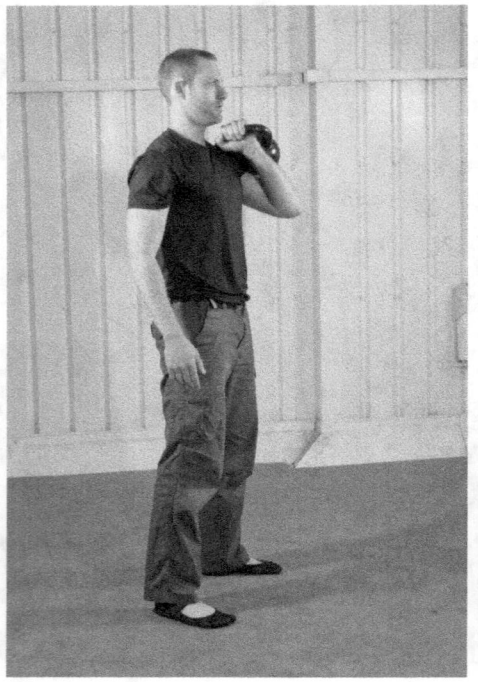
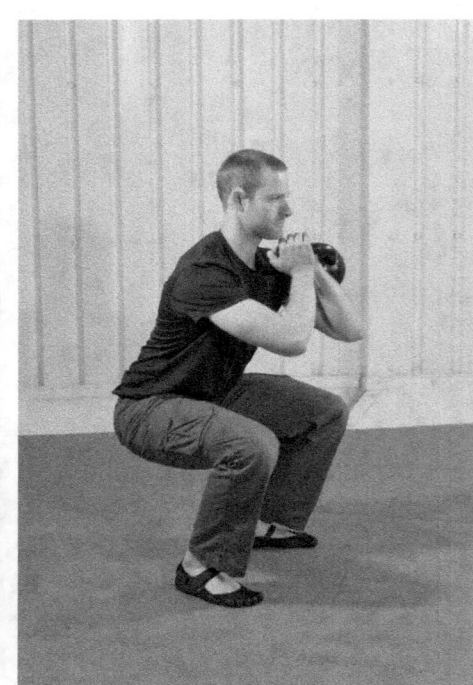
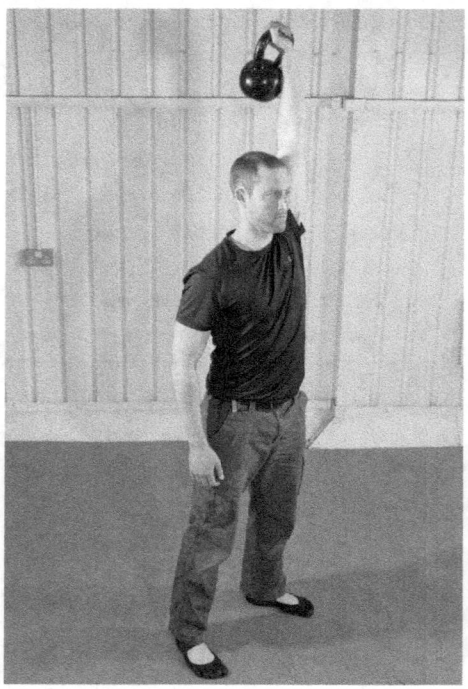

1. Set your posture (shoulders down, head up, glutes tight, abs tight).

2. Raise the kettlebell up to your chest and rest it on your biceps.

3. Stand with your feet slightly wider than shoulder-width apart and pointing forwards.

4. Push your hips backward.

5. Push your knees forwards towards the outside and front of your feet.

6. Keeping your chest high sit down on an imaginary chair.

7. Go as deep as you can while maintaining a straight back (in conjunction with your hip stretch this will improve the more you do).

8. Drive your hips forwards and use the momentum to press the weight overhead.

9. Return the kettlebell to your chest and repeat as directed.

Single arm clean

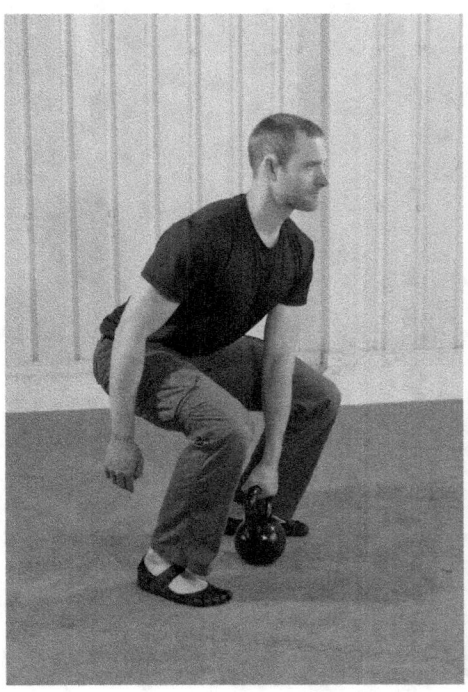 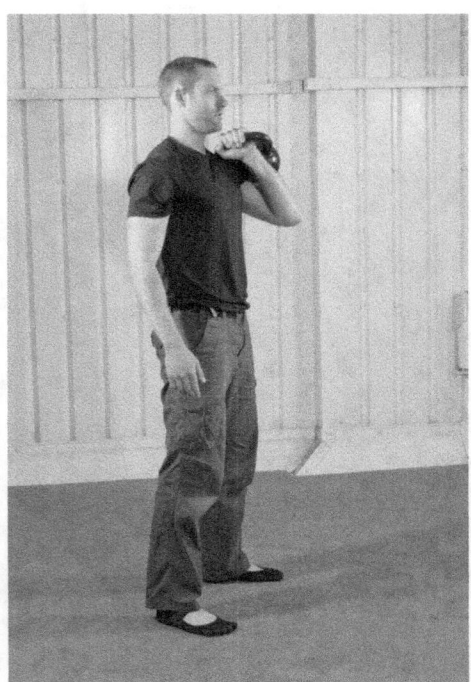

1. Set your posture (shoulders down, head up, glutes tight abs tight).
2. Extend hips back, bend knees and take hold of kettlebell.
3. Ensure your back is straight.
4. Lift the weight and slowly stand.
5. Once the weight reaches your knees drive hips forward like a kettlebell swing.
6. Pull the weight and rotate the kettlebell.
7. Use the momentum to guide the kettlebell into a resting position on your upper arm.
8. Repeat as advised.

I highly recommend finding the video for this technique http://absolute-health.co.uk/exercise-demonstrations//

Single arm clean to press

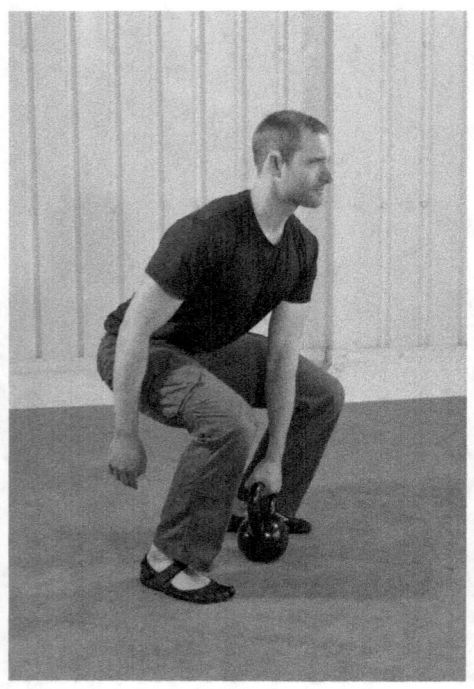

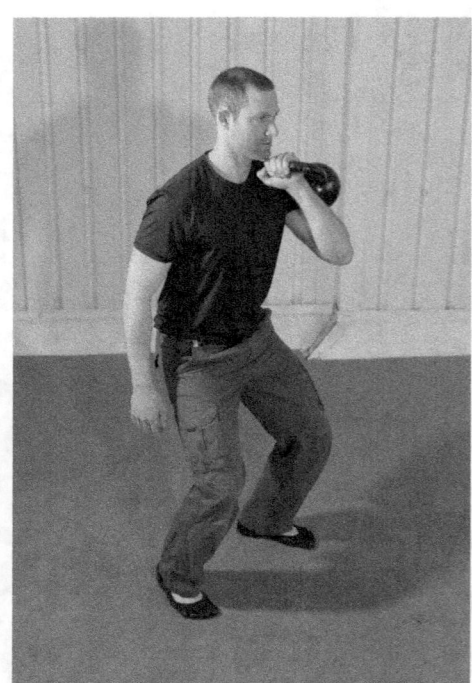

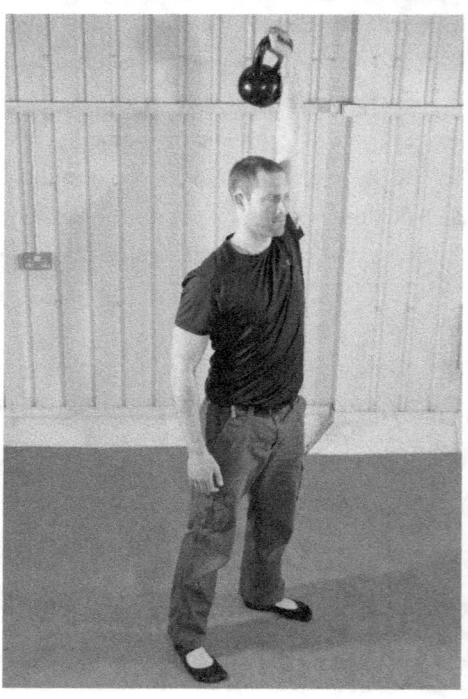

1. Set your posture (shoulders down, head up, glutes tight, abs tight).
2. Maintaining all postural cues, extend hips back and bend knees.
3. Take hold of kettlebell.
4. Ensure your back is straight.
5. Lift the weight and slowly stand.
6. Once the weight reaches your knees drive hips forward like a kettlebell swing.
7. Pull the weight and rotate the kettlebell.
8. Use the momentum to guide the kettlebell into rest on your upper arm.
9. Cushion the catch by bending your knees slightly.
10. Drive upwards and press the kettlebell overhead.
11. Repeat as directed.

I highly recommend finding the video for this technique http://absolute-health.co.uk/exercise-demonstrations/

Single arm kettlebell swing

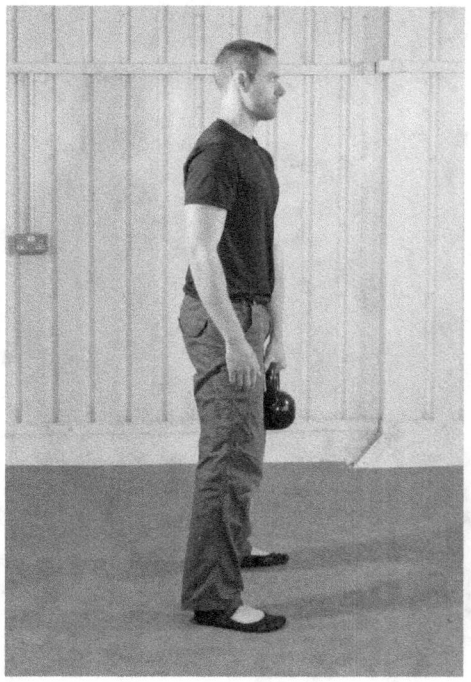
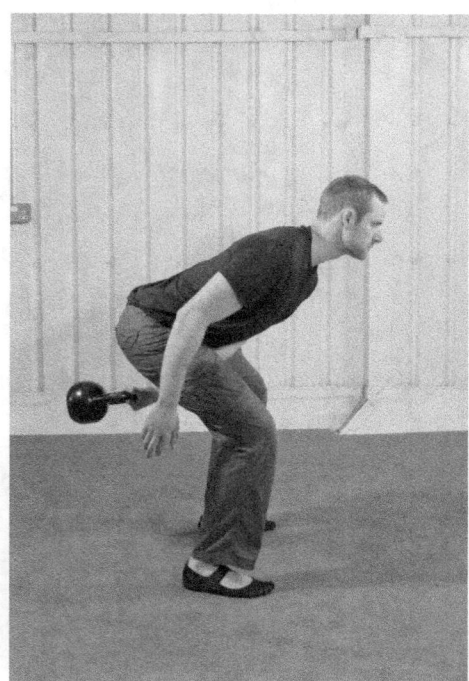

1. Set your posture (shoulders down, head up, glutes tight, abs tight).
2. Push hips backwards and relax your arms.
3. Set hips as far backwards as you can and swing kettlebell back.
4. Drive your hips forwards as if you are trying to jump forwards.
5. Allow kettlebell's movement from the hips to arc the weight upwards
6. As the kettlebell reaches the top of the arc your body should be in set posture position
7. As kettlebell falls, sit your hips back again.
8. Repeat as directed.

Visit http://absolute-health.co.uk/exercise-demonstrations/ for video demonstration

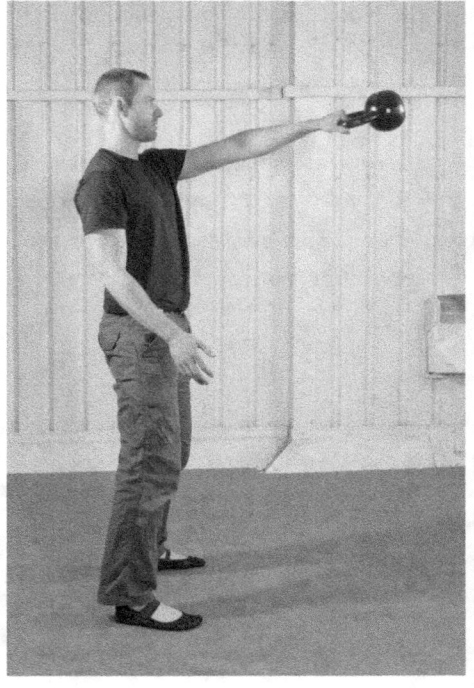

Single arm deadlift

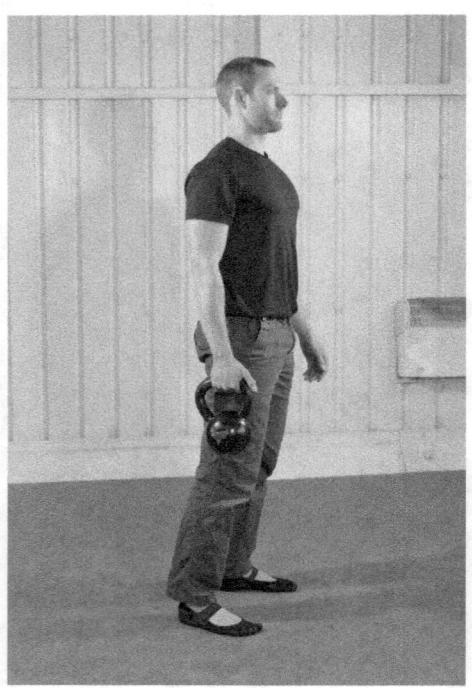 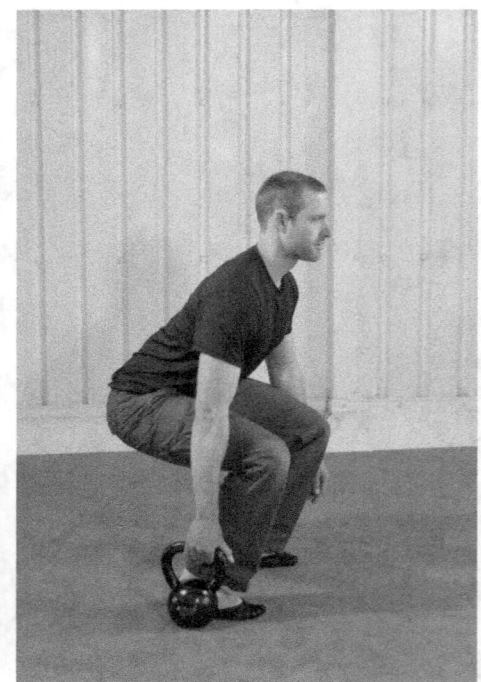

1. Set your posture (shoulders down, head up, glutes tight abs tight) with weight on the floor next to your ankles.

2. Sit your hips backwards until your hand reaches the kettlebell.

3. Lift your chest and ensure your back is straight.

4. Drive your hips forward returning to set posture.

5. To lower weight, sit your hips backwards until kettlebell reaches the floor.

6. Try and stablise your core to ensure movement symmetry.

7. Repeat movement.

Single arm bent over row

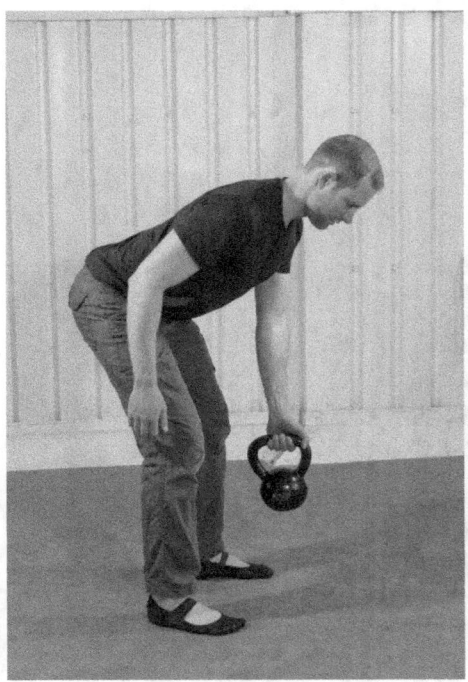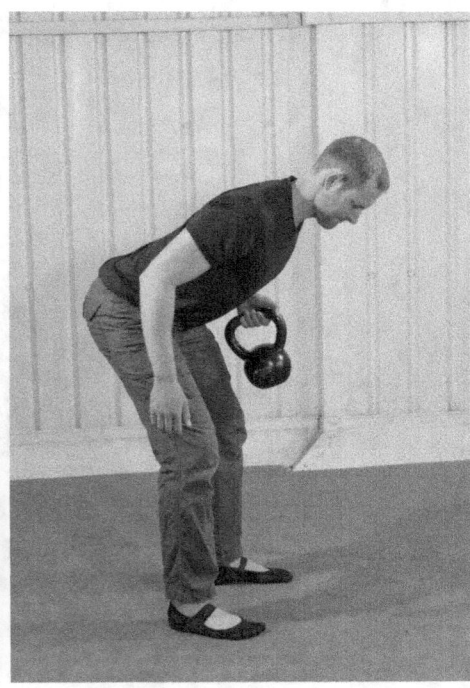

1. Set your posture (shoulders down, head up, glutes tight, abs tight).
2. Push hips backwards to bend forward (you should feel a hamstring stretch).
3. Reassess all postural cues, apart from glutes.
4. Pull weights up, pushing your elbow towards your hips and squeeze shoulder blades together.
5. Keep shoulder squeezed as you lower the weights under control to a straight arm.
6. Maintain posture and avoid rotation.
7. Repeat as recommended.

Chest press

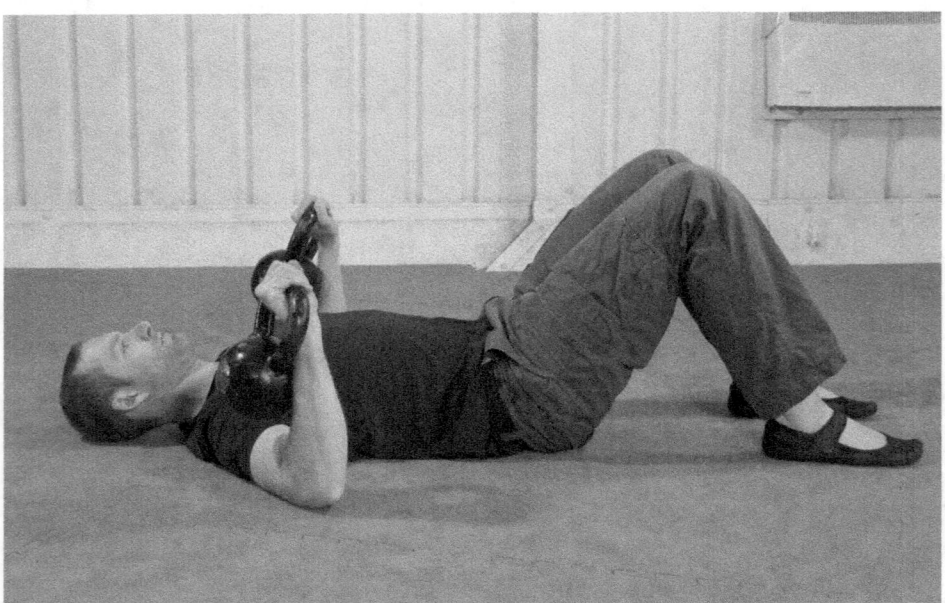

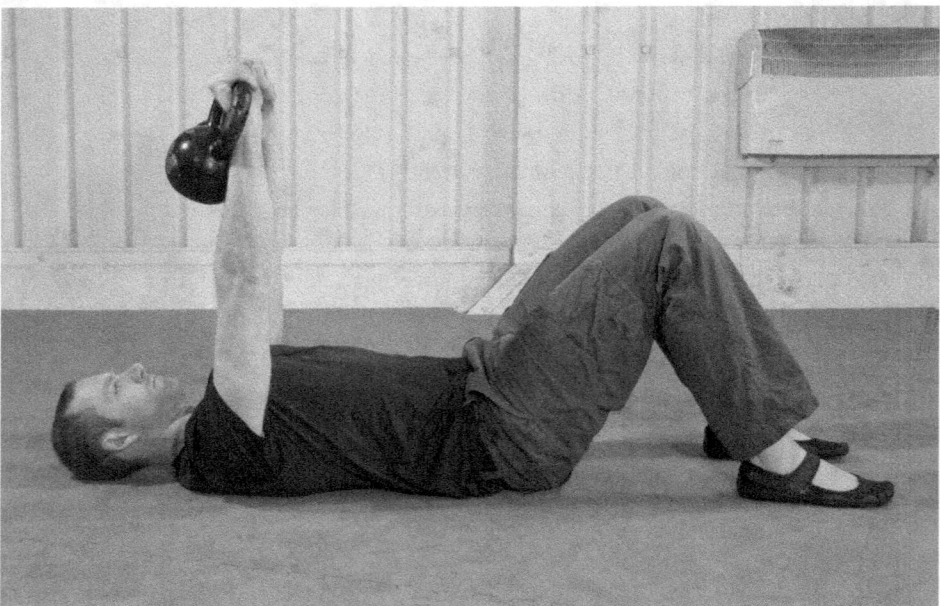

1. Set your posture (shoulders down, glutes tight, abs tight).
2. Hold the kettlebells in your hands, place your wrist above your elbows with your elbows at 70 degrees to your body.
3. Imagine the kettlebells are on a bar and you are trying to bend that bar as you press the weights up directly above your shoulders.
4. Straighten arms at top of the movement.
5. Repeat as recommended.

fitfor.biz

Single arm chest press

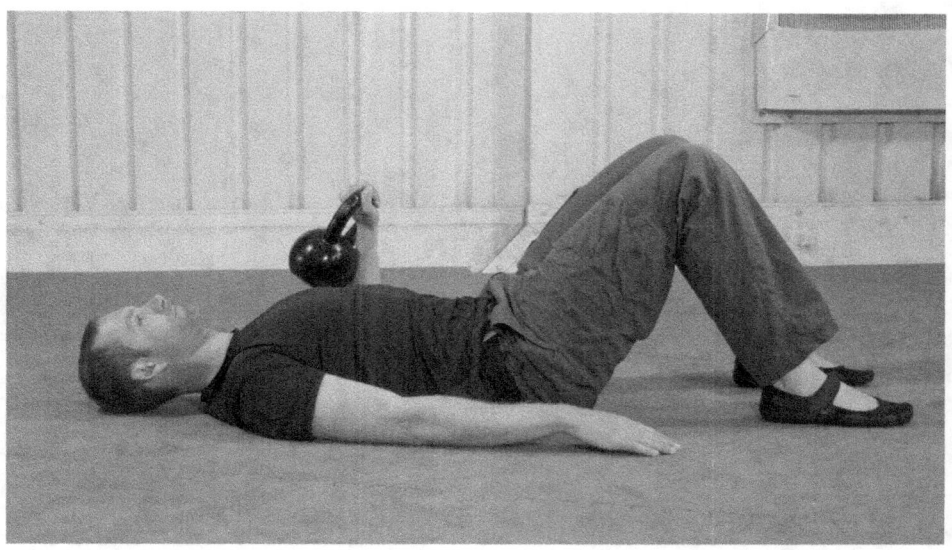

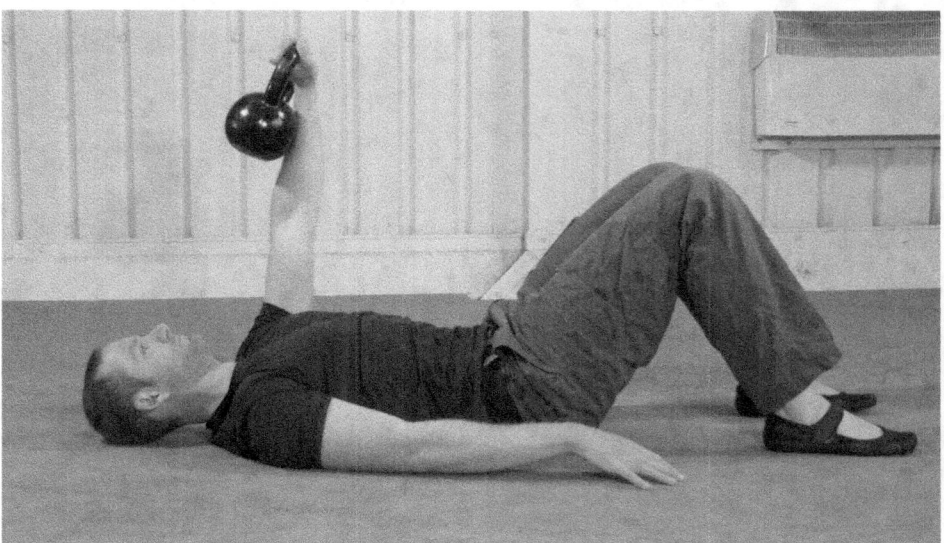

1. Set your posture (shoulder down, head up, glutes tight abs tight).
2. Hold the kettlebells in your hands, place your wrist above your elbows with your elbows at 70% to your body.
3. Imagine the kettlebells are on a bar and you are trying to bend that bar as you press the weights up directly above your shoulders.
4. Straighten arms at the top of the movement.
5. Brace core to fight rotation.
6. Repeat as recommended.

Kettlebell press up

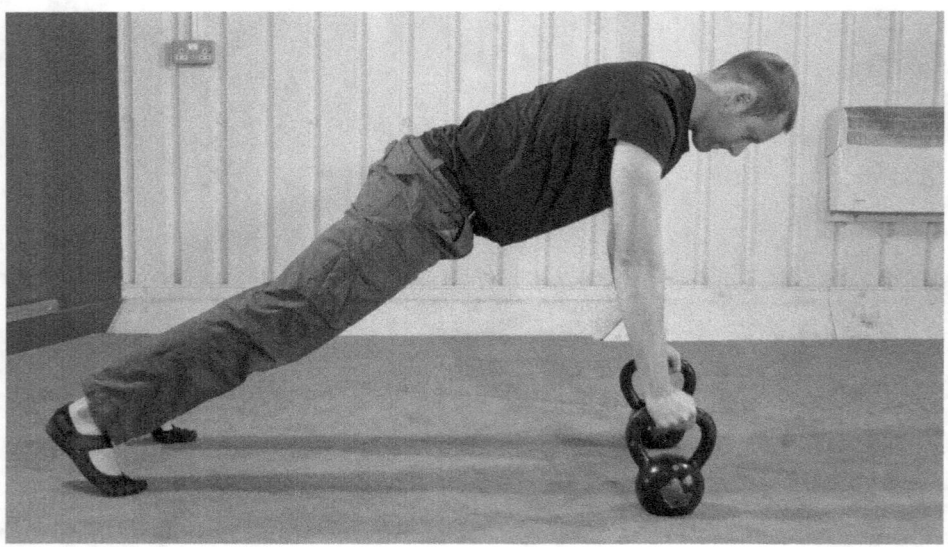

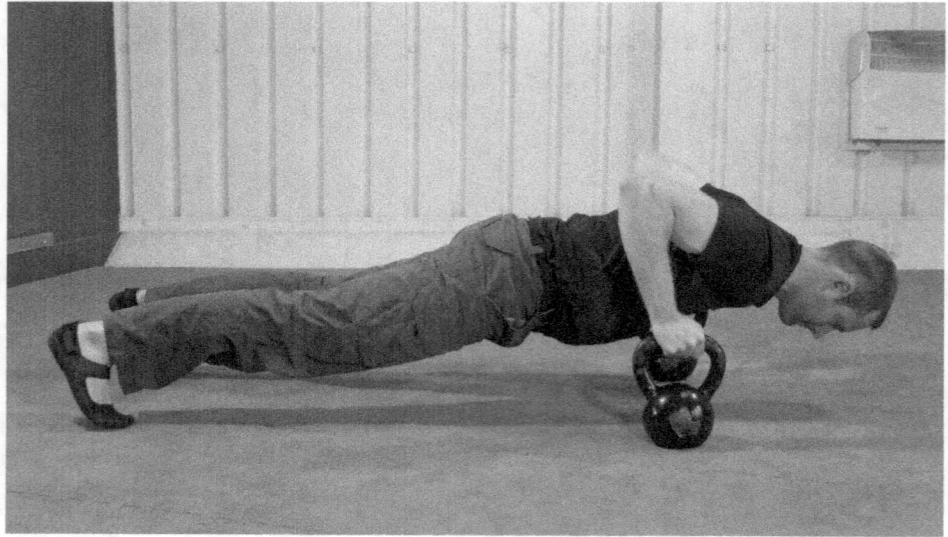

1. Assume the press-up position, then set your posture
2. Place hands slightly wider than shoulders.
3. Maintaining set posture, lower your body towards the floor.
4. Place feet together.
5. Rotate hands outwards so palms are almost facing each other.
6. When your nose reaches the floor, push up through the heel of your palm.
7. Keep elbows above wrists.
8. Repeat as recommended.

Romanian Deadlift

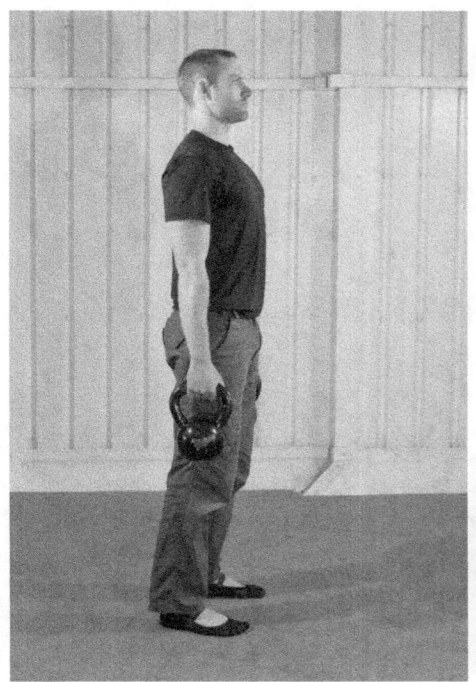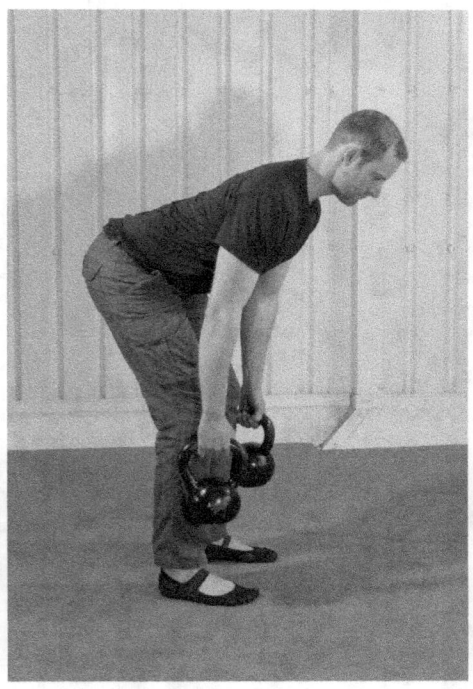

1. Set your posture (shoulders down, head up, glutes tight, abs tight).
2. Push hips backwards to bend forward (you should feel a hamstring stretch).
3. Reassess all postural cues apart from glutes.
4. Drive your hips forward to return to postural set position.
5. Repeat as recommended.

Single arm Romanian Deadlift

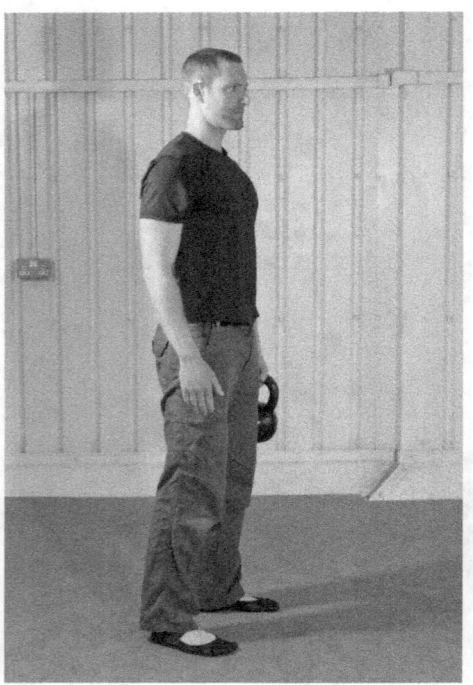 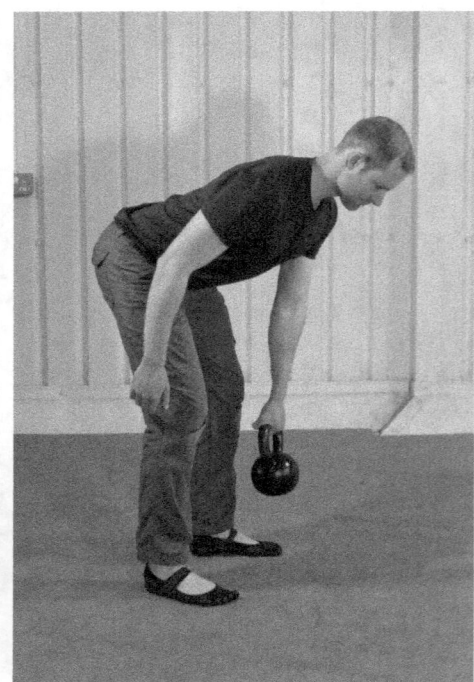

1. Set your posture (shoulder down, head up, glutes tight, abs tight).
2. Push hips backwards to bend forwards (you should feel a hamstring stretch).
3. Reassess all postural cues apart from glutes.
4. Drive your hips forward to return to postural set position.
5. Maintain posture to avoid core rotation.
6. Repeat as necessary.

Single arm snatch

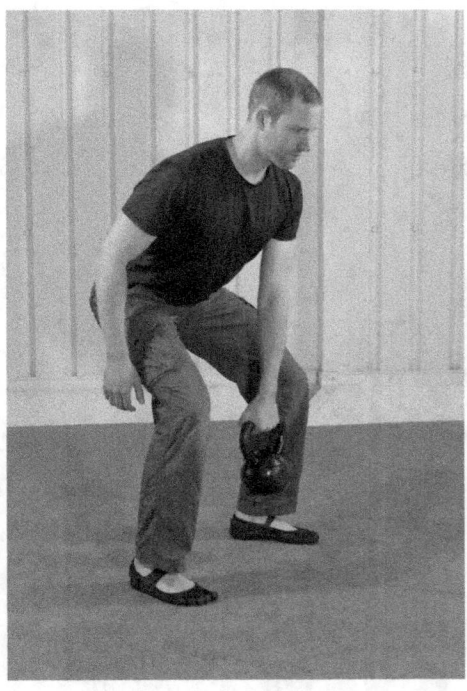 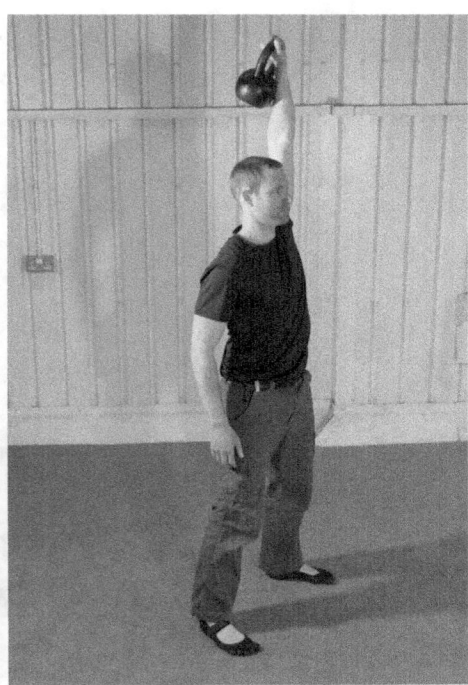

1. Set your posture (shoulders down, head up, glutes tight, abs tight)
2. Push hips back and slightly bend knees.
3. Hold hands level with knees.
4. Drive hips forward and guide kettlebell overhead.
5. Flip kettlebell over and bring to rest gently on your wrist.
6. Repeat as directed.

This move requires good timing and should be perfected with a light kettlebell to avoid injury. I highly recommend following the video http://absolute-health.co.uk/exercise-demonstrations//

Turkish Get up

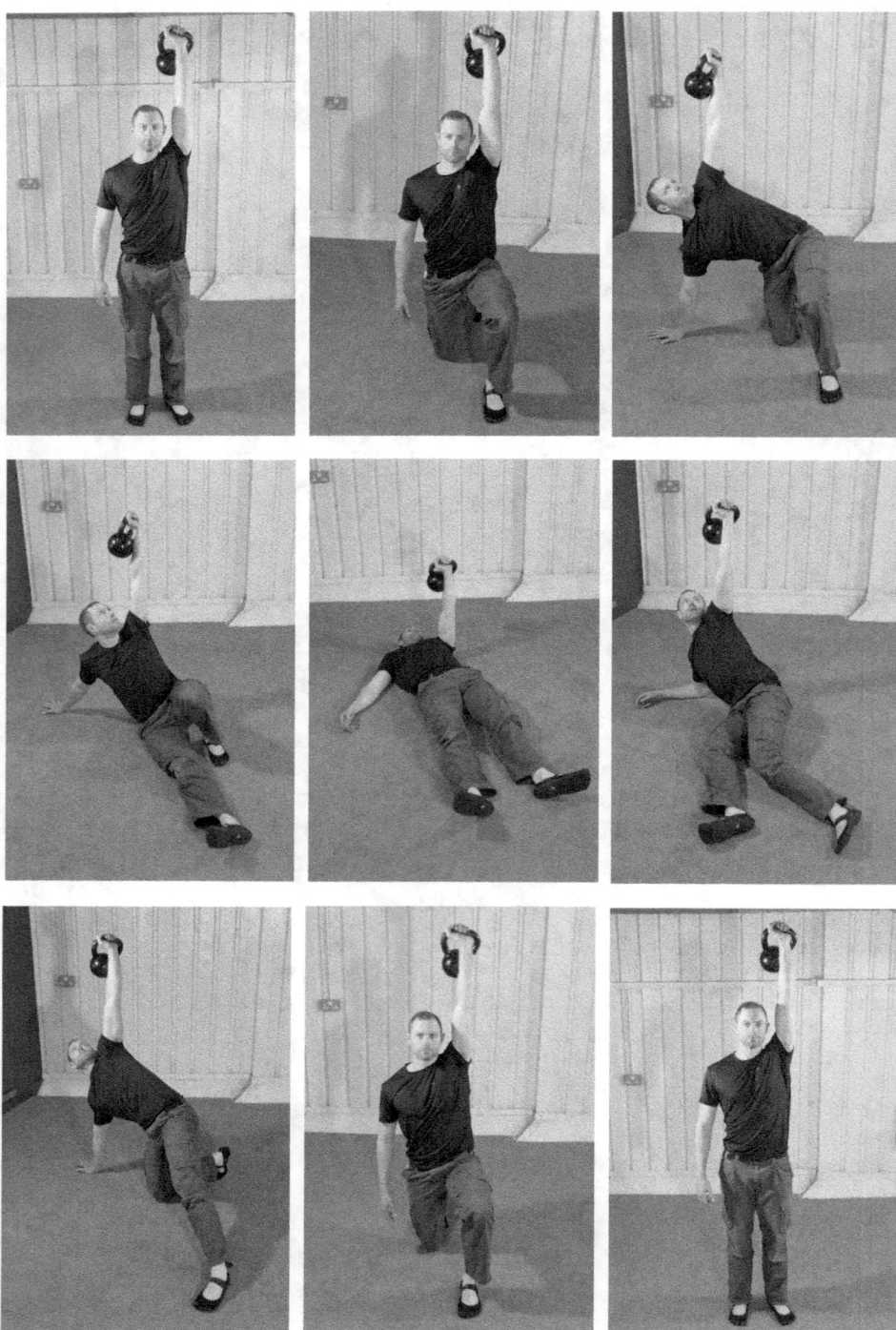

The workouts

At this point I should re-iterate that movement is a skill and not something that needs to be forced. As long as you maintain time constraints and effort levels progress, intensity and fitness will all follow.

If you complete a workout and you are able to maintain good posture throughout with little rest then increase load, reps or intensity or upgrade to the next workout. I will provide eight workouts. If you complete each workout two/three times a week for three/four weeks with necessary progressions, they should last you for months. At this point, you can either look to go back to the earlier workouts and increase intensity or construct your own.

Either way you will be a skilled kettlebell-user and in much better shape than you are today.

These workouts are pretty intense and are designed to be completed without rest. The idea behind these workouts is that they will build strength, muscle, muscle endurance, posture, core stability, postural strength while burning fat and improving cardiovascular fitness. A big ask but absolutely achievable.

Tabata

As with any fitness regimen in the real world, success is determined by the ability to continue during the most stressful and busy times. With that in mind, Tabata workouts provide a useful base and are only four minutes long.

Treat these as your introduction to training. Everyone has time for a four-minute workout before getting ready in the morning and setting the alarm four minutes earlier should be something achievable.

You will no doubt be thinking that 4 minutes cannot make a difference. However, if you are new to regular exercise, but even if you're not, Tabata is the perfect incubator from which to experience and monitor the dramatic effects that it can have on your life with regards to fitness, energy and vitality throughout your day.

It will also help you progress in fitness while you are in the movement learning phase of training. Use this as your base level of training: don't have time for a full session? Do a Tabata.

Tabata is 20 seconds of effort followed by 10 seconds of rest x 8

Options include:

Running, rowing, skipping, star jumps, hill climbs, burpees, squats, lunges, kettlebell swings.

For your first week, insert into your day planner (URL TK) three Tabatas on Monday, Wednesday and Friday.

For your second week, insert I Tabata every morning.

The workouts

Each time you complete a workout insert weights used, number of sets completed and number of reps completed next to the recommended

Rep: individual exercise repetition, e.g. 1 squat is 1 rep.

Set: complete set, e.g. 10 squats is 1 set.

Workout 1

Exercise Circuit	reps	sets	date kg	date kg	date kg	date kg	date kg	date kg	date kg
Backward lunges (both sides)	10	4							
Walkouts	5	4							
Chair single-arm row (both sides)	10	4							
Bridges	10	4							

Workout 2

Complete as many sets as you can in 15 minutes

Exercise Circuit	reps	sets	date kg	date kg	date kg	date kg	date kg	date kg	date kg
Body weight squats	20								
Bent over row	10								
Press-ups or knee press-ups	15								
Deadlifts	10								

Workout 3

Exercise Circuit	reps	sets	date kg	date kg	date kg	date kg	date kg	date kg	date kg
Kettlebell squats	10	4							
Dead row (both sides)	8	4							
Push press	8	4							
Kettlebell swings	15	4							

Workout 4

One set of left-side exercises plus burpees, followed by one set of right-side exercises set plus burpees equals one set

Exercise Circuit	reps	sets	kg	date time	date time	date time	date time	date time	date time
Single arm deadlift	8	3							
Dead row (both sides)	8	3							
Single arm chest press	8	3							
Burpees	10	3							

Workout 5

Exercise Circuit	reps	sets	kg	date time	date time	date time	date time	date time	date time
Single arm squat (both sides)	10	4							
Single arm clean (both sides)	10	4							
Single arm push press (both sides)	10	4							
Single arm swing (both sides)	10	4							

Workout 6

Exercise Circuit	reps	kg	date time	date time	date time	date time	date time	date time	date time
KB squat to press	30,20,10								
Burpees	30,20,10								

Workout 7

Exercise Circuit	reps	sets	date kg	date kg	date kg	date kg	date kg	date kg	date kg
Turkish get-up	5	5							
Single arm Romanian deadlift (both sides)	10	5							
Weighted squats	20	5							

Workout 8

Exercise Circuit	reps	sets	date kg	date kg	date kg	date kg	date kg	date kg	date kg
Single arm snatch (both sides)	8	6							
Single arm clean to press (both sides)	8	6							
Kettlebell press-ups	10	6							

Chapter 6

Productivity and self

Manage your state

The decisions we make on a day-to-day basis make up the sum total of who we are. The reason we create new habits designed to push us towards our goal is to limit our decisions, leaving energy to make the right decision when it's important.

Even when we have built up habits, stress can get on top of us and override the habit - especially new ones which can be fragile. The reason behind this is that decision-making is state dependant. This means that when we are anxious, tired, stressed, hungry, angry, excited; we make our decisions based on these emotions.

This not only relates to important work decisions but it ties together all parts of this book: making the decision not to go to bed because you must find out who gets voted off The X Factor; deciding not to go to the gym because you are busy; making poor food choices to instantly gratify your hunger. These decisions are led by your emotion of the moment. Anger is probably the easiest way to highlight this. Have you ever had an argument with someone you love and said something you instantly regretted? At the root of this is a decision made that was based on emotion. When you're not in an argument your rational brain makes the decision that next time you fight you will back down to keep the peace. Unless you create a strategy for dealing with this situation your reaction will continue to be the wrong one because your response will always be chosen during a moment of high stress, based on the emotion you are experiencing at the time.

While anger is a great example, the fact is that in a much less noticeable way our state affects every decision we ever make. This impacts not only big obvious decisions but far more importantly the small decisions. Should I check my email or finish what I am doing? Should I chat a bit longer or get back to work? Should I focus on the task that will have the greatest impact on my business or should I do a load of small low-impact jobs in a bid to feel productive? These are the sort of questions that determine our success, productivity and overall life satisfaction. The following section is designed to elevate your state helping you to make better decisions, while giving you the tools to increase your productivity in all areas of your life.

Habits are the first defence here as they allow you to make rational decisions in advance. Your nutrition programming, sleep times and workout times have become habitual. They will soon be processes that require little thought at all. The next stage is to find other areas of your life that can become habitual.

It should be noted that everyone has different stressors. The youngest of three children is unlikely to see any elevation in stress as a result of a conflict. Likewise, the military are trained to manage stress levels during confrontation. Learning to manage situational stress then is an important part of the equation, especially if you frequently find yourself in situations that increase stress and anxiety. Our life experiences go a long way to creating our particular stressors: an only child for example might see any disagreement as a sign of attack and become defensive (if you're an only child reading this you're no doubt thinking 'no I don't').

Task 1

People have been writing for years about the secret to happiness but very little has been proven to permanently elevate mood, although it does seem that two people can have exactly the same experience and exactly the same feelings but remember it very differently. How we frame our physiological responses to situations seems to have a huge impact on our happiness.

I was speaking to my coach, Michael, who told me this great story to illustrate my point:

Michael was speaking with a friend about roller coasters. He was saying how much he loved them…not even just the ride but the build-up, "it's just so exciting". His friend then said how much he hated them. "I can't stand the build-up, my palms sweat, my stomach starts doing summersaults, I just feel so anxious", he said. 'Oh that's how I describe excitement", Michael said.

How we frame our memories and experiences has an impact on our mood and writing seems to be one thing that can significantly boost our state. A study by Pennebaker, Kiecolt-Glaserand Glaser (2004) found that students who wrote about their traumatic experiences for 15 minutes every day for four days showed an improvement in immune function. In a study conducted by Emmons and McCullough (2003), subjects improved their level of happiness by 25% simply by sitting down and writing five things they were grateful for.

If it wasn't already clear your task is to write before you go to bed: five things that went well during your day; and two things that could have gone wrong but didn't. This will also help to build a positive association with your day. I like to use the app 'Day One' but pen and paper works just as well and I won't tell anyone you keep a diary!

Task 2

In 1988 a study conducted by Strack, Martin and Stepper discovered that we can literally trick ourselves happier. It turns out that mother does know best; putting a smile on your face will cheer you up! During the study, one group of participants were told to hold a pencil sideways in their mouths forcing their muscles to replicate a smile position. The other group were told to hold the pencil between their lips, forcing a frown. Both groups were then sat down to watch cartoons.

The smile group reported a more intense humour response. It seems that we each have our own set happiness level that is expressed outwardly. In order to change, your set level requires a constant reminder of what your face is doing.

Your task here is of course to smile more. Think more 'secret smile' than 'Dick Van Dyke'; a massive grin is not necessary. I find a great way to do this is to combine it with the postural re-adjustment exercise (which will also elevate mood and confidence).

I use the app Chime for this, a nice lady tells me the time every 15 or 30 minutes and I reset my posture and check if I'm smiling yes, (I am aware how ridiculous this sounds). In your mind, you are no doubt thinking that you are going to look crazy.

Don't worry, it naturally fits into your day and nobody will even notice you are doing it. This book has nothing in it that I haven't done myself or had others do without great results. If you were to take on daily task away from this book I would recommend it be this one.

Set goals

In the beginning of all change there is a place we wish to be and a place we have been. The interesting thing about visualising goals is that while it is one of the best things you can do, it is also one of the worst things you can do.

To begin with we must visualise the completion of our goal, paying special attention to what we will gain from it and how it will feel to achieve it. From here, we can create a series of action steps in order to lead us to completion of the task.

However, the problem with vivid and frequent visualisation of what we will gain from achieving our goal is that it robs us of our motivation. If the secret to happiness to be content with what you have then you can use this method but using this method can remove your drive to achieve you goal. Teaching your mind how to experience what you will receive upon the completion of a task is vital but, doing so too frequently will trick the brain into thinking it has already achieved its goal.

My goal in writing this book is increased credibility and being considered as an expert in the field of long-term health change. This will lead to greater success; which in turn will lead to more time with my family. The visualisation of more time with my family is being on holiday and relaxing with my family around me and the joy and contentment I feel in that moment. In order to motivate myself to complete the huge task of writing a book I summon the visualisation of what I will achieve by writing this book. This is useful during times of low motivation to re-ignite the spark and remind you of why you are doing what you are doing.

Your task is to visualise what you will gain from completion but only once a week, you could even write it down.

Impact bias

Again, both helpful and harmful, awareness of impact bias will help you to avoid it. We are designed to accomplish things; our brain's drive is to further our genetics. The more successful we are, the greater its chances of doing this.

Our brains drive us to complete goals by creating a perception that goal achievement will make us happier than it actually will. I frequently see it in my gym with muscle gain or fat loss clients. Improved self-image may come through improved physique and there are a million other reasons for getting fit and healthy. Goal achievement is not however the direct route to happiness that our brains can sometimes convince us it is. Obviously there are positives to this effect: it can help us to believe that goal achievement will bring happiness. If we didn't believe this we would never do anything.

A really common story is the tale of the successful person who has everything they ever wanted and has found that it didn't bring happiness. This person is clearly driven and this comes from a strong perception of what goal achievement will bring. Unfortunately, what goes hand in hand with an inflated perception of what success will bring is the inevitable disappointment when each time a goal is achieved the previously anticipated reward isn't there.

The **TOTE** model is a great model for highlighting the process of successful goal completion:

- Test
- Operate
- Test
- Exit

Success often follows this model. Successful people will continue to test and operate until a successful test condition is achieved and the exit can be taken. It is also worth noting that success is only achievable with repetitive and measured failure. Thomas Edison followed this exact model in his attempt to create the light bulb. He tested, then operated, then failed and returned back to the start while noting what didn't work. He repeated this system 999 times before reaching the exit point. This model is only usable, however, when we have taste. If we take 'The X Factor' as an example: the two types of people we like the most are the 'Susan Boyle's' (the normal-looking, even slight misfits with the voice of an angel) and those who get up and produce a noise like a drowning cat and yet have no idea how bad they are. The second type is lost. They are unable to chart their progress and improvement as a singer as they have no taste; they have no knowledge of where they are on their journey to becoming a singer. The singer who knows they are bad, however, is who we want to be. Visualisation of what the end will bring us becomes hugely important when we have had an afternoon of screeching. Success comes from knowing where you are, knowing where you have been and knowing where you are headed.

The majority of the time needs to be spent in the now. Happiness is then derived from seeing how far we have come, not in the feeling of arrival.

Use your goal to get you back on your feet and turn your attention back to the task at hand. Each time you complete a test phase, be aware that you are now a different person to the person you were at the start of the test. Awareness of your progress is where meaning is found.

Be mindful of your own evolution and know that goals are a stepping stone on an ever-moving end point. The evaluation of how far you have come is then more valuable than looking at where you are. A proper assessment of where you actually are to begin with can help. Measuring yourself against your peers is a surefire way to make you the best of a bad bunch. Whatever your goal is make sure you have a full, independent and honest review of where you are now, along with markers that will demonstrate progress.

Progress in the beginning of most goals with focus, whether related to business, health, learning a skill will come quickly. If you are learning the violin, for example, you will most likely learn each note quite quickly, and combining two will follow soon after. After a while though you might reach a plateau which might knock you off your stride, it could derail you completely.

Having the ability to look back and see how far you have come can be enough to push you back into the progress phase again.

Task:

Set goals. This can be done for health, business, family and friends. Try setting three for each. Write them down:

Health:

Business:

Family:

Friends:

Now for each visualise what you will gain by achieving your goal. Make it vivid, really experience how it makes you feel. Now step back out of your visualisation and reveries and map what needs to happen in order to complete each goal. This is now your to-do list. Focus on getting each step done in order.

- Once a week re-visualise why you are pursuing your goal.
- Once a week look back at what you have done.
- Now refocus on your list.

Increase your focus

I used to pride myself on keeping on top of my email, my calls and my texts; sometimes I was so in the zone I'd be juggling 10 conversations at the same time, doing the business accounts and giving a comprehensive breakdown as to why someone on the Internet is wrong. There is no doubting that I felt productive but after a couple of months I started to notice two things.

Although I was busy I wasn't producing anything and I was pressing refresh on my iPhone like a rat with a cocaine dispenser. I very quickly learned two lessons; being busy and productive are two different things, and the only way to reduce your emails is to send fewer.

I resolved then to stop being busy and start being productive. The first point of action was to stop being a slave to email. I had a look around the internet at email productivity ideas and the best idea I found was to answer emails in the afternoon and tell my clients that I was doing this with an auto responder.

I have heard a number of people have had great success with this method; where it fails for me and many of my clients is that they need to be contactable to move appointments or to have pressing questions answered.

Another simple idea for email reduction is the phone. Mark emails that are conversation starters and ring them, encourage clients to call you rather than email, quite often a 20 email conversation can be saved with a 5 minute phone chat.

Email might be quick and simple but it creates email. If you have questions for people fight the temptation to put a tick in your done column and do all of your calls in the 3pm lull. Most people have an energy low around 3pm and will welcome the chance to chat rather than focus on a screen.

This next one does not work for many but a public diary can really help make you organise your time better and help remove the appointment booking emails.

Finally the system that I use for getting more work done and keeping my focus away from email and text is called Pomodoro. Pomodoro is like interval training for the mind. It involves high intensity bouts of focus followed by measured rest periods.

Popularised by Tim Ferriss in this book The Four Hour Work Week, Pomodoro hides its genius in its simplicity. It aids in focusing on one specific task while applying just enough time pressure to create the urgency that we often require to get things done.

The best way to get tasks completed quickly is to give them your sole focus but without a time frame it is too easy to allow distractions to creep in, after all you have all the time in the world to get your work done or at least a deadline that is far enough away that you're yet to feel its pressure. Once we get used to working an 80 hour week it start to become our norm and productivity drops during times of low pressure.

Pomodoro is also really useful for showing us how long tasks take us. There aren't many of us who can say we know how long it takes us to complete the things we do from day-to-day. With Pomodoro it becomes easy to measure our productivity and therefore easier to manage our time.

Task

Choose a task from your list, it could be reading, it could be writing a document, but it should be something that you can complete without the assistance of anyone else. Prepare your environment for work. This could mean putting your phone on silent or out of easy reach if you need to accept calls. It could mean using Internet or social media blockers. Try to find a place where you won't be disturbed.

Now, set a timer for 20 minutes. Apply singular focus to the task and get to work. Use the last minute to note:

- How much did you get done (word count perhaps)?
- Did you achieve singular focus? If not, what distracted you and what will you do differently next time?

Now the important part: set your timer for 10 minutes' rest. Check your emails, go and get a coffee, read my latest article on Facebook, have a chat with a colleague or make a call, do your postural exercises. Make sure you are back at your desk and ready to start your next 20-minute block.

Once you master the 20-minute/ 10-minute intervals for a number of hours you can look to prolong your working time. This will depend largely on how much of this sort of work you have to get done. Always remember to be strict with your working and resting times. Without the time pressure we lose focus easily.

Learn to fail and fail fast

In 2009 the recession hit and Gordon Ramsay, along with the rest of us, went through some difficult times. His restaurant Amaryillis was all over the papers, it was going through some hard times. It turns out that during a global recession people are less likely to have as many extravagant dinners, especially in Scotland.

There was an opportunity here to tell a story of how Gordon was weathering the storm and successfully turned his business around; instead he was annihilated by the media. This is not a stand-alone story, rather one that perfectly demonstrates the media's intentions to create a culture of fear. Fear of failure sits on this list.

The media's portrayal of failure permeates through our society and is evident in everything we ever do. School punishes failure with regular gradins, not in just tests but in day-to-day work. By the time we leave school, fear of failure cripples our entire lives and it's visible everywhere we look: in relationships we should have let fail, in businesses we should have let go - or the reverse - in adventures, new relationships and new businesses that we are too scared to start for fear of failure.

We need to learn to appreciate the value of failure. The person who has failed 1000 times is in a better place to succeed as long as they learn the lessons that failure holds.

If we make this specific to our goal of health and performance, fear of failure could be our greatest enemy. We know that there are numerous factors that could derail our cause. Eating cake is a good example. Our fear of failure pushes us to create series of 'don'ts' in our mind: in this case 'don't eat cake'.

Unfortunately, the mind does not process a negative well, we think in images. For example, if I say 'don't think of a purple elephant' your mind instantly creates an image of a purple elephant. In the same way, when we say 'don't eat cake', our mind instantly creates an image of cake. Probably the best cake in the world. When you have visualised cake in this scenario you have already failed. Your mind will now create a situation in which you will eat cake by producing neuropeptide Y which increases carbohydrate cravings. If not cake, it will be something that produces the same feedback as cake. When we eat high carbohydrate (sugar) foods, our brain produces serotonin. Serotonin increases calm and gives us a feeling of contentment and well-being (that 'ahhh' feeling we get after high carbohydrate food). This an in-built neurological response created at birth. Whenever we cried as a baby we were given breast or bottled milk, a high-carbohydrate, high-protein comforter. So the narrative we create in our mind in order to avoid failure is the very thing that makes failure unavoidable.

Task

Change your narrative. We learn by metaphors and stories, the stories we tell ourselves and others become truths very quickly. We can use these stories to make failure less likely.

'I only eat bread every once in a while'

'Cake affects my performance so I tend to avoid it'

'The rewards I get from eating cake are outweighed by the negative effects'

Everyone has stories that hold them back in many areas. If you can isolate those stories and change them it will have a hugely positive impact on your life.

Some common examples:

'I'm rubbish at x so I don't do it'

'I have no willpower'

'I only have to be near someone sick for a second and I get ill'

'I'm so weak'

'I'm so fat'

Task 2

Optimise your comfort. Comfort eating is ingrained we cannot avoid it. If you tell yourself not to eat something you are creating a fetish. **You have become the crazy person smoking in the aeroplane toilet.** Eating that comfort food that you love is going to happen, so make sure you optimise the experience.

Eat your comfort food the way a wine taster drinks wine. Eat slowly, sumptuously, and mindfully, respect the treat.

You will eat less of it. The goal with a treat is to eat, not have eaten.

Task 3

T

O

T

E

Every new experience is open to failure. The faster you fail and the more comfortable you become with failure, the more success you will have.

Follow the above acronym with every new task. Only move to exit once the task is mastered or complete.

Learn what you are already doing

By our very nature as business people, we are addicted to our to-do list; tick after tick builds momentum, we just want to get more and more work done. Sometimes we start the day with a few wins and we find ourselves in 'the zone'.

The zone or 'flow state', as psychologist Mihály Csíkszentmihályi called it, is a state in which you are mentally fully immersed, enthusiastic and focused on what you are doing. We all fall into this state from time to time but, learning to create it is the key to productivity.

The art of creating this flow is having a clear runway ahead of you; knowing what you need to do and exactly what needs to happen next in order to continue moving forward in your flow. Having to stop and work out what needs to happen next and jumping from one task to the next is a sure way to keep yourself out of flow state. In order to create flow state you need a detailed but flexible to-do list that produces daily tasks in order of importance. This helps to keep your list small and allows you to work in order of priority rather than in order of which task you would prefer to do.

Task I

Start your week with one to two hours' planning. Just like changing your health, productivity is all about planning. List all the projects that you are working on or wish to work on. Now, working backwards, list all of the individual things that need to happen in order to complete each project. Put a note or a name next to any of the tasks that need to be done by someone else as these can be quickly out-sourced.

Thanks to the wonders of modern technology, there are some great websites and apps that will drip-feed tasks to you in order of priority.

I personally use www.getitdoneapp.com. I have ten ongoing projects and ten constantly changing weekly tasks, yet I am emailed each day with just three or four things I need to do. Focusing on just one task at a time really helps me to concentrate on what I am doing and get into flow state almost every day.

Task 2

There are things that we do on a regular basis that can be outsourced, cut out or done more efficiently, there's even dead time that could be used more effectively. The trouble is, we have no idea what those things are or when that time is. This is a much easier task than it appears to be and I have seen it gain some people from five to ten extra hours per week.

Print out a full-day diary and every 15 minutes write down what you did in the previous 15 minutes. You will be amazed at how you are able to claw back time. For example, studies have shown that if we step away from a task temporarily onto another, it will take on average 20 minutes to regain focus on the first task. A good way to illustrate this would be taking a break from preparing a document to check emails quickly. Structuring a time in your day when you do your emails would be a much more efficient use of time.

I would recommend avoiding emails in the morning as your day will be reactive as opposed to proactive. Tasks that are done two or more times a week and done exactly the same every time can be taught to someone else and outsourced. Similarly, if a task does not require your specific skills and it can be done by following a simple system then it can be outsourced.

People often find that they spend more time on the road than is necessary. Driving in rush hour, for example, or driving to use services, such as the gym, where an alternative exists closer. It's not until we see the compound interest on paper that we can see the full picture. If you can find 20 minutes a day, you will have saved a 70-hour week over the course of a year.

Time invested in your health is not wasted time; time wasted working inefficiently is. You cannot get time back; you can only make sure you don't waste any more.

Learn to be happy

During Shaun Anchor's brilliant TED talk he referred to his time spent at Harvard studying students in order to learn about happiness. He noted that a friend had asked, 'what do students at Harvard have to be unhappy about', alluding to the obvious privilege in which they live. Shaun said that 'embedded in that question is the key to understanding happiness'.

He went on to share details from his research:

If we know everything of someone's external world, we are only able to predict 10% of their happiness. Ninety percent of our long-term happiness is predicted not by our external world but by the way our brains process it.

Twenty-five percent of job success is predicted by IQ, 75% of job success is predicted by our optimism, our social support and our ability to see stress as a challenge rather than as a threat.

Psychologist Mihály Csíkszentmihályi described two different types of memory:

The semantic memory. This is our story, our life narrative, it is how we make meaning of things. It is who we believe we are.

The procedural memory. Procedural memory is like muscle memory, this is when we are performing repetitive actions that we are very good at, this is where flow occurs.

The semantic memory and the procedural memory are unable to function at the same time. If we are telling ourselves a story then we are inhibiting our brains ability to enter procedural memory. In order to go into procedural memory we must temporarily suspend the story of 'you'.

As a child we rarely have time in flow unless we have perhaps become particularly competent in a certain sport. You will remember as a child that days and weeks felt incredibly long. This is from not being in flow.

You will also remember days more recently where you lost track of the day, you got to work then suddenly it was time to go home. Csíkszentmihályis describe this as 'time out of mind'. As we get older and much of what we do becomes habitual, we spend more time in flow.

Flow is where life satisfaction comes from; getting things done that have meaning to us.

Respected neuroscientist Antonio Demasio says there are two kinds of emotion: your base and your reaction.

Winning the lottery would create a spike in happiness. Similarly, being sacked from your job would create despair but both emotions would be fleeting. Your level of happiness before both these events occurred would be your base level. Winning the lottery wouldn't create a permanent lift in happiness levels.

Let's take orgasms as another example: if someone was born experiencing permanent orgasm, they would be the only person in the world who didn't know what an orgasm felt like. Orgasm would be the base level.

If we could assign an arbitrary number to both positive and negative effects, let's say 6. If our base level is 0, then when we experience something amazing we hit a 6 and when we experience something bad then we hit -6. If our base level is -3 though, then anything good would only take us to a 3, whereas a bad experience would take us to -9 before we returned to our negative base level.

The key to life satisfaction then - or happiness, if you want to call it that - is to elevate your baseline. This is done through accomplishment and mindfulness; that is to be mindful of your past accomplishments.

Task

Meditate on your life in cycles, this does not mean to sit cross legged and squeeze thumbs and forefingers together and say "om" (unless you want to). It simply means that once a week you should give thought to what you have accomplished and visualise what you wish to accomplish before returning to now.

Too much time spent in the past will encourage you to rest with what you have, too much time in the future will convince you that you already have what you want. Excellence and accomplishment will raise your baseline.

Take a step back and see what you have, remind yourself of a time where that was all you ever wanted.

When I wake up in the morning and look across at my beautiful wife, I consciously remind myself of a time when waking up to a beautiful woman who is fun to be around was all I ever wanted.

Seeing what I now have through the eyes of someone who wants it more than anything has the effect of making me more grateful, more romantic and prevents me from taking what I have for granted.

Thanks for reading

Ask a teenager today to imagine a world without the internet, mobile phones and social media; ask them if they think they could live in it. Ask them to describe what it would be like and they don't have a clue. These things have dramatically impacted the lives of many that remember a time when they didn't exist.

Those who grew up with it, however, have no frame of reference; asking them to imagine a world without these things is asking them to imagine a world that has never existed. Imagining a day is completely different from a lifetime, almost every aspect of life is slightly or dramatically different as a result of this technology.

This effect is repeating over and over with each new generation.

Today we have no possible way of imagining a world without computers or without lights or without electricity.

From remote controlled televisions to cars and computers, each new invention that storms the globe has to answer one question: does it save the user time and effort?

The list of time saving inventions that have appeared in the last 100 years is huge. Unfortunately the vast majority of us use this extra time in order to spend more time in the office rather than more time at play. We end up working longer hours, facilitated by overhead lighting so that we can afford more or better quality time saving inventions.

Today, more so than any other time in human history, we have to go out of our way to be healthy. Our lives are created around a system that is designed to keep us at our desks and entertained for as many hours as possible.

Throughout human history, being free from disease by simply living our lives was enough to keep us incredibly fit and healthy. Fitness and health is now more than ever a choice and the more difficult one at that.

As pack animals we are driven to be the same as those around us but imitation in today's world is often a recipe for poor health. Following the crowd is no longer an option.

If your goal is to be the best, to accelerate past your competition who are solely focused on the hours they put into their work then this is your silver bullet.

Use this book.

Create a plan.

And prepare to become truly limitless.

References

Colpo, A. (2012) *The fat loss Bible*. (p. 41). 1st Ed. converted to ebook by wordzworth.com.

Baumeister, R.F. and Vohs, K.D. (2007) *Self-regulation, ego depletion and Motivation*. (p.16) Social and Personality Psychology Compass, Florida State University, University of Minnesota.

Pilon, B. (2008-2009) *How much protein*. (p. 39). 1st Ed. Strength Works Inc.

Pilon, B. (2012) *Eat Stop Eat*. (p.41). 1st Ed. Ontario Canada: Strength Works Inc.

Murnahan, B. (2010) *Stress, Anxiety Reduction due to Writing Diaries, Journals, Emails, and Weblogs*. (p. 109). Eastern Michigan University.

Duhigg, C. (2012) *The Power of Habits*. (pp. 12-13). 1st Ed. Great Britain: William Heinemann.

Mah, C. (2008) *Ongoing Study Continues to show that Extra sleep improves athletic performance*. (p. 9). American Academy of Sleep Medicine. [available at: www.sciencedaily.com] [accessed: August 2012].

Kresser, C. (2010) *When it comes to fish oil, more is not better*. (p. 37). [available at: Chriskresser.com] [accessed: June 2013].

Csikszentmihalyi, M. (1990) *Flow - The Psychology of Optimal Experience*. (p. 111). Haper Collins publishing.

Anderson, D.E. Ph.D. (May 2013) *The National institute of Aging*. (p. 29) [available at: www.grc.nia.gov/branches/crb/danderson.htm] [accessed: May 2013].

Dr Ratey, J. and Hagerman, E. (2009) *Spark How exercise will improve the performance of your brain*. (p.58). 1st Ed. Great Britain: Clayd Ltd, St Ives plc.

Dr Starrett, K. (2013) *Becoming a Supple Leopard*. (exercise section) (p. 71-98). 1st Ed. USA: Victory Belt Publishing Inc.

Dawson, D. and Reid, K. (1997) *Fatigue, Alcohol and performance impairment nature*. (p. 8) Vol 388, July 1997. HBR.ORG.

Lenneville, E (2013) *Why do I think better after I exercise?* (p. 58). Scientific America.

Cook, G. (2010) *Movement functional Movement Systems*. (Exercise section) (p. 63). 1st Ed. Aptos, CA: On Target Publications.

Hotting, K. and Roder, B. (2013) *Beneficial effects of physical exercise on neuroplasticity and cognition*. Pub Med. [available at: Pubmed.gov] [accessed: May 2013].

Vrenken, H. et al (2008) *Reduced Orbitofrontal Parietal Gray Matter in Chronic Insomina*. (p. 27). Frontiers in Neurology. [available at: www.sciencedirect.com] [accessed: May 2013].

Foucault (1978) *The History of Sexuality*. (p. 22) Vol. 1: An Introduction, 1st Ed. Random House Inc.

Ferrie, J.E. et al (2007) *A prospective study of Change in Sleep Duration: Associations with Mortality in the Whitehall II Cohort*. [available at: www.journalsleep.org] [accessed: May 2013].

Kim, S.J. et al (2011) *Relationship between weekend catch-up sleep and poor performance on attention tasks in Korean adolescents*. (p. 29). Department of Psychiatry, Gachin University of Medicine and Science, Rebublic of Korea. [available at: Pubmed.gov] [accessed: May 2013].

King, L .A. (2001) *The health benefits of writing about life goals*. (p.114). Personality and Social Psychology Bulletin, (798-807). [available at: Pubmed.gov] [accessed: April 2013].

Labi, H, et al (2013) *Increase risk of coronary heart disease among individuals reporting adverse impact of stress on their health*. European Heart Journal, 216(10). [available at: eurheartj.oxfordjournals.org] [accessed: June 2013].

Layman, D.K. (2004) *Protein quantity and quality at levels above the RDA improves adult weight loss*. Department of Food Science and Human Nutrition, University of Illinois USA. [available at: Pubmed.gov] [accessed: May 2013].

Stone, L. (2008) *Just Breathe: Building the case for Email Apnea*. (p. 23). [available at: The Huffington Post] [accessed: www.huffingtonpost.com].

McDonald, L. (2007) *The Protein Book A Complete Guide for the Athlete and Coach*. (p. 39). 1st Ed. Salt Lake City: Lyle McDonald Publishing.

Sisson, M. (2009) *The Primal Blueprint*. (p. 54). 1st Ed, Malibu, CA: Primal Nutrition inc.

Moss, Micheal (2013) *The Extraordinary Science of Addictive Junk Food*. (p. 53). The New York Times, 20 February.

Tomporowski, P.D. (2009) *Exercise and Children Intelligence, Cognition, and Academic Achievement*. Pub Med. [available at: Pubmed.gov] [accessed: April 2013].

Wolf, R. (2010) *The Paleo Solution*. (p. 45). 1st Ed. The United States: Victory Belt Publishing.

Smolensky, M. (2001) *The body clock guide to better health*. (p. 31) Henry Holt and Company llc.

Andreas, S. and Faulkner, C. (1996) *NLP The New Technology of Achievement*. (p. 104). 1st Ed. London: Nicholas Brealey Publishing London.

Strack, F., Martin, L.L., and Stepper, S. (1988) *Inhibiting and facilitating conditions of the human smile: a nonintrusive test of the facial feedback hypothesis*. (p. 113). American Psychological Association. [available at: Pubmed.gov] [accessed: April 2013].

Perry, S. (2012) *Right here, write now* (p. 113). [available at: www.psychologytoday.com] [accessed: March 2013].

Wiley, T.S. and Formby, B. Ph.D. (2000) *Lights Out*. (p. 28) 1st Ed. USA: Pocket Books.

Wahls, T.L. (2011) *The seventy percent solution*. Pub Med. [available at: Pubmed.gov] [accessed: Jan 2013].

Ferriss, T. (2011) *The 4 hour work week*. (p. 109). 1st Ed. United States: Vermilion Imprinted of Ebury Publishing A Random House Company.

Tkach, C. (2005) *Unlocking the treasury of human kindness: Enduring improvements in mood, happiness, and self-evaluations*. (p. 112), Unpublished doctoral dissertation, University of California. [available at: spring.org.uk] [accessed: Dec 2013].

Willett, W.C. (2013) *Promotion and selection by serum growth factors drive field cancerization, which is anticipated in vivo by type 2 diabetes and obesity* (p. 8) Proc. Natl. Acad. Sci. USA: 13927-13931.

Wu, H. et al (2010) *Effects of different sleep restriction protocols on sleep architecture and daytime vigilance in healthy men*. Dept. of Neurology, Insititute of Neuroscience, Neurosicence Research Centre of Changzheng Hospital, Shanghai, PR China. [available at: Pubmed.gov] [accessed: Nov 2013].

Youngstedt, S.D. et al (2013) *Chronic moderate sleep restriction in older long sleepers and older average duration sleepers: A randomised controlled trail*. Dept. of Exercise Science, University of South Carolina, Columbia, US. [available at: Pubmed.gov] [accessed: June 2013].

www.ingramcontent.com/pod-product-compliance
Lightning Source LLC
Chambersburg PA
CBHW060413290526
45791CB00002B/734